Practical Vascular Technology: A Comprehensive Laboratory Text

NATHALIE GARBANI, Ed. D.(c), H, RVT

Vascular Sonography Program
Nova Southeastern University
Fort Lauderdale, Florida

  Wolters Kluwer | Lippincott Williams & Wilkins
Health

Philadelphia · Baltimore · New York · London
Buenos Aires · Hong Kong · Sydney · Tokyo

Acquisitions Editor: Peter Sabatini
Senior Product Manager: Heather Rybacki
Associate Product Manager: Kristin Royer
Marketing Manager: Allison Noplock
Manufacturing Coordinator: Margie Orzech-Zeranko
Typesetter: Macmillan Publishing Solutions
Printer & Binder: C&C Offset Printing

First Edition

Copyright © 2010 Lippincott Williams & Wilkins, a Wolters Kluwer business

351 West Camden Street　　　　530 Walnut Street
Baltimore, MD 21201　　　　　　Philadelphia, PA 19106

Printed in the United States of America

9　8　7　6　5

Library of Congress Cataloging-in-Publication Data
Garbani, Nathalie.
　Practical vascular technology: a comprehensive laboratory text / Nathalie
Garbani. – 1st ed.　p. ; cm.
　Includes bibliographical references.
ISBN 978-1-58255-809-7 (alk. paper)
1.　Blood-vessels--Diseases--Ultrasonic imaging.　I. Title.
[DNLM: 1.　Cardiovascular Diseases–ultrasonography. 2. Ultrasonography–methods.
WG 141 G213p 2010]
RC691.6.U47G37 2010
616.1'307543–dc22

2009034727

DISCLAIMER

Care has been taken to confirm the accuracy of the information present and to describe generally accepted practices. However, the authors, editors, and publisher are not responsible for errors or omissions or for any consequences from application of the information in this book and make no warranty, expressed or implied, with respect to the currency, completeness, or accuracy of the contents of the publication. Application of this information in a particular situation remains the professional responsibility of the practitioner; the clinical treatments described and recommended may not be considered absolute and universal recommendations.

The authors, editors, and publisher have exerted every effort to ensure that drug selection and dosage set forth in this text are in accordance with the current recommendations and practice at the time of publication. However, in view of ongoing research, changes in government regulations, and the constant flow of information relating to drug therapy and drug reactions, the reader is urged to check the package insert for each drug for any change in indications and dosage and for added warnings and precautions. This is particularly important when the recommended agent is a new or infrequently employed drug.

Some drugs and medical devices presented in this publication have Food and Drug Administration (FDA) clearance for limited use in restricted research settings. It is the responsibility of the health care provider to ascertain the FDA status of each drug or device planned for use in their clinical practice.

To purchase additional copies of this book, call our customer service department at (800) 638-3030 or fax orders to (301) 223-2320. International customers should call (301) 223-2300.

Visit Lippincott Williams & Wilkins on the Internet: http://www.lww.com. Lippincott Williams & Wilkins customer service representatives are available from 8:30 am to 6:00 pm, EST.

Preface

This manual was conceptualized and designed around one main goal: to provide a practical approach to diagnostic vascular sonography (this term is used for consistency throughout the manual even though several of the technologies and techniques described do not involve the transmission of sound). The vision throughout the development of this manual was that it would find its audience spread from students to more accomplished sonographers and be an easy-to-use reference for techniques and interpretation of data. As such, the manual focuses on pictures, diagrams, algorithms, and concept maps to introduce, explain, and enhance the understanding of the process and procedures involved in presenting information for diagnosis of vascular diseases.

The educational philosophy of the manual was based on the concept of meaningful learning using a strong visual approach in sequential, logical steps. In such context, the text has been kept to a minimum, mostly through captions of the images and diagrams illustrating the concepts and essential points developed in each part and chapter. The underlying idea of meaningful learning is to promote critical thinking based on the acquisition of essential basic concepts with the intent of progressive integration of these concepts within each particular situation. Patients are highly individualistic in their backgrounds, risk factors, presentations, prognosis, and expectations. Each exam is a new adventure to be lived through a close team approach between a patient, a sonographer, a referring physician, and a treating physician. This manual will provide road maps to successfully assist the members of the team.

Remaining true to the goal and educational philosophy of this manual, the author has taken great care to avoid expressing strong personal opinions or bias based on experience. Indeed the author has based concepts, facts, and ideas on an extensive literature search to reflect the state of knowledge and research in the field of vascular diseases. The readers are therefore strongly encouraged to obtain some or all of the referenced sources and forge their own opinions. The author gracefully recognizes that protocols differ from one setting to another, as they should to reflect and be tailored to the patient population, the equipment used, and the expertise and comfort of all members of staff. The author hopes that this manual provides at least some information relevant and/or useful for all.

As an educator, the author recognizes the importance of the partnership in teaching and learning between educators and students, senior and novice sonographers, and sonographers and physicians, and hopes that this manual will build this bidirectional bridge.

Acknowledgments

First and foremost, my thanks go to my parents Huguette and Jean-Pierre Garbani and my daughter Natacha. Without their support and understanding, none of what I have accomplished would have been possible. They gave me the space, the time, and more importantly the emotional support I needed to move forward with my projects (this being one of many). I would also like to thank a dear friend and colleague Samuel Yoders for his insights and support.

I am grateful to all those who participated in my training as a vascular technologist over the years and who therefore contributed in more ways than they may know, or that I even acknowledged, in leading me here today. In a chronological fashion, they are:

1. Drs. Alda Cosi, Karl Beckman, and Chris Molgaard, as well as David Weinstock and David Smith (who by now are probably physicians, but who were then technologists);

2. Drs. James Menzoian and the late Jay Coffman who gave me the chance to lead my first lab, (with David Smith still at my side for some time), as well as Drs. Jonathan Woodson and Albert Hakaim;

3. Drs. William Clutterbuck and Patrick Mahon, who greatly embody integrity and patient dedication in the field of vascular surgery;

4. Colleen Danault, office manager, who taught me almost everything in billing and coding, and much more;

5. Drs. Isaac Mehrez, Arman Kasparian, Frederick Bartlett, and Frank Vittimberga, who appreciated my clinical skills and judgments in addition to my technical skills.

Of course my path was also made possible by many others—friends and some adversaries (the world is not always a big friendly place!), patients, and support staffs—who challenged me, appreciated me, or criticized me, and I thank you all.

These special thanks would not be complete without acknowledging the contribution of all my students for all past 5 years, as well as Dr. Richard Davis, dean of the College of Allied Health and Nursing at Nova Southeastern University. And last but not least I would like to thank the staff of Lippincott Williams and Wilkins, Wolters Kluwer, without whom I may not have undertaken such a project.

Introduction

For ease of use, the manual is divided into four parts representing major arterial and venous territories: the head and neck, the upper extremities, the abdomen, and the lower extremities and the pelvis. Each part is further divided in chapters representing the major areas of testing encountered in a dedicated vascular laboratory. The chapters are constructed around general concepts for each testing modality, tips and rationales for the exam, algorithms or decision trees, and detailed step-by-step explanations, through visual displays of patient preparation, testing sequence, and results and interpretation. Each chapter or section closes with summative tips to enhance, emphasize, or add to the concepts discussed previously.

Intended to offer a practical approach to vascular sonography, the manual does not present a dedicated section or chapter on physics concepts. Many experts have published comprehensive books on ultrasound physics, and attempting to summarize their work in a chapter would not give justice to the content needed but, most importantly, would be beyond the scope of this manual.

Therefore, it is strongly recommended that the reader be familiar with physics and hemodynamics concepts, at all times, not just when reading this manual, because the work done in a vascular laboratory could not be complete without a thorough understanding of the underlying technology.

Furthermore, although this introduction will focus on some general concepts in pathology and therapy, these will remain mostly in the form of reviews of published works and studies. This manual will not provide basic or fundamental concepts in physiology or pathophysiology. Just like physics, these would be beyond the scope of this manual and the expertise of the author. It is therefore recommended that the readers be familiar with basic science concepts and/or substantiate the practical information with other readings and references.

This introduction will be dedicated to important and general concepts to be used throughout the manual and related to:

- The role we play as vascular sonographer in the health care team,
- The representation of the data we obtain through ultrasound and other physiologic tests, and
- How to present the data in light of:
  - The particular context and condition of the patient,
  - The present state of knowledge of pathologic processes affecting the circulatory system,
  - The therapeutic possibilities.

Role of the Vascular Sonographer in the Health Care Team

While the field of vascular technology may seem restricted in its scope, the individual patient embodies an array of functioning systems that can rarely, if ever, be isolated from the other physiologic systems or the psychosocial or spiritual environment. This concept, used thousands of years ago in ancient Egypt by the healer Imhotep (1, 2) and Maimonides (3), is regaining strength as a more comprehensive medical model.

Figures 1 and 2 illustrate this point and will serve as a basic tool for assessment of each component of the vascular system. The concept is that a patient presenting with a set of symptoms should be considered within his/her social context, his/her medical and familial history, his/her inborn characteristics, and his/her demographics. All these factors can have a different impact on the symptoms but also can have a significant impact on the testing, prognosis, and treatment. Although the role of vascular technologists or sonographers is legally restricted to acquiring information, the reality is that as a part of the interdisciplinary health care team and as an expert in a specific field, this role cannot be taken in the sole context of equipment operator. Therefore, vascular sonographers need to be involved in answering the same questions as physicians, which are:

1. Are the symptoms consistent with a vascular condition? If not, can we safely rule out such possibilities or offer some insights into other potential underlying problems?

2. If the symptoms are linked to vascular pathologies, where are the most serious problems, how severe are they, and how will the condition and the potential therapy affect the patient's quality of life?

3. What can be done about the condition?

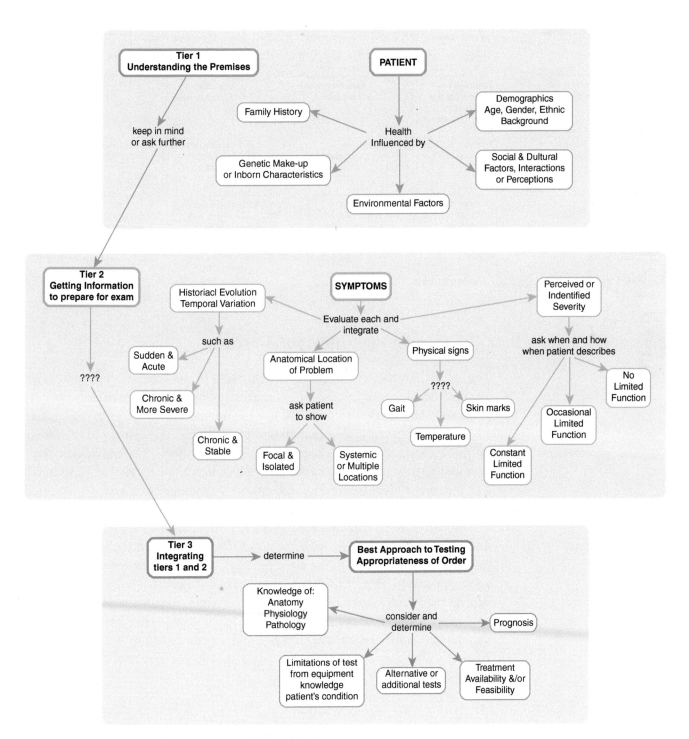

FIGURE i.l   Integration of information, thinking globally.

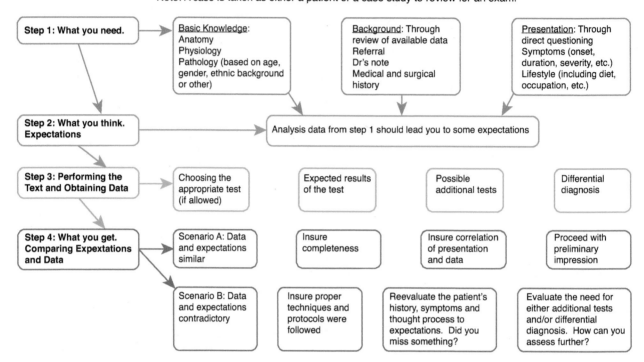

How to Think Through a Case In Vascular Ultrasound

Note: A case is taken as either a patient or a case study to review for an exam.

FIGURE i.2   Proceeding through a vascular case.

Understanding Data Displayed on an Ultrasound Screen

The following section will pertain exclusively to the formation of images on an ultrasound screen in relation to anatomic and transducer orientation. As previously stated, this section will not include details on physics principles.

Unlike other technologies in diagnostic imaging, the display of the image on the ultrasound screen is highly operator dependent. The transducer position and approach relative to the targeted structure to be viewed, displayed, and measured must be clearly understood by the operator *and* documented for the interpreting physician.

By convention, it is assumed that the patient is in an anatomic position and the transducer is held with the notch directed toward the head in a longitudinal approach and to the right of the patient's body when using a transverse approach. This convention should be followed to assure that images can be read and interpreted correctly by anyone *and* in the absence of the sonographer who obtained the data. Any changes from this convention should be annotated on the images and documented in the preliminary report.

Patient/Transducer Positioning

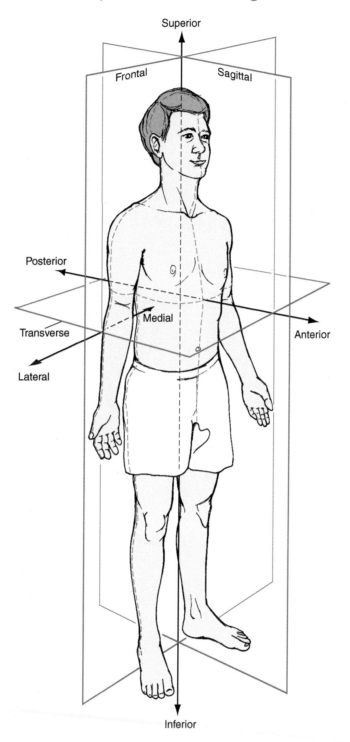

FIGURE i.3 Conventional anatomic position and anatomic planes.

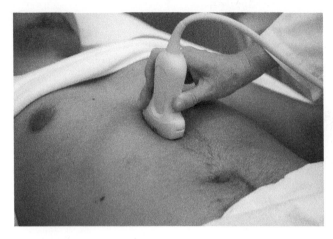

FIGURE i.4 Anterior approach of the abdomen in sagittal or longitudinal.

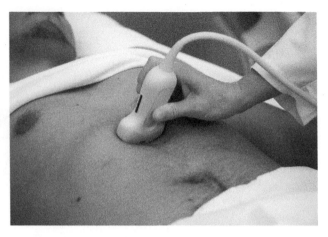

FIGURE i.5 Anterior approach of the abdomen in transverse.

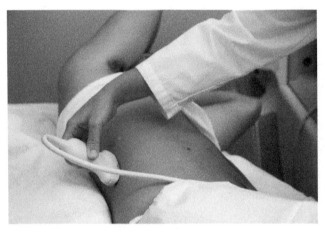

FIGURE i.6 Lateral approach of the abdomen in longitudinal.

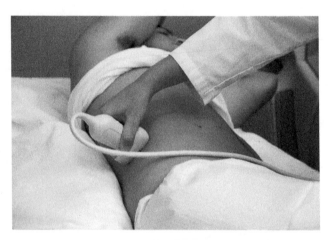

FIGURE i.7 Lateral approach of the abdomen in transverse.

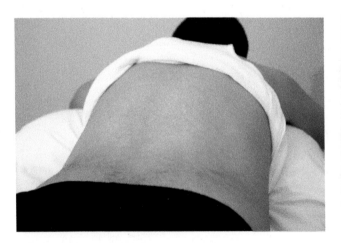

FIGURE i.8 Patient prone.

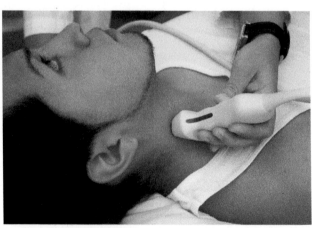

FIGURE i.9 Anterior approach of the neck in longitudinal.

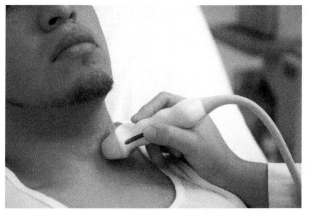

A

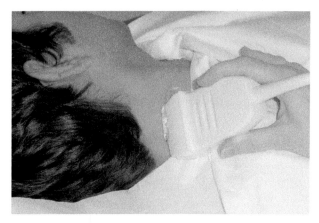

B

FIGURE i.10   Anterior (A) and posterior (B) approach of the neck in transverse.

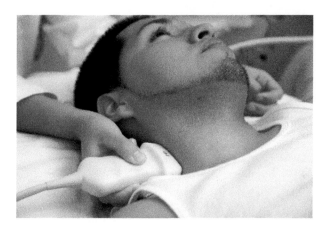

FIGURE i.11   Posterior approach of the neck in longitudinal.

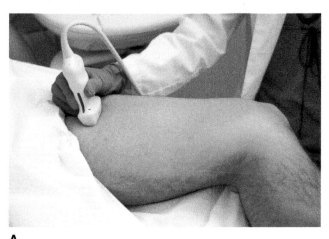

A

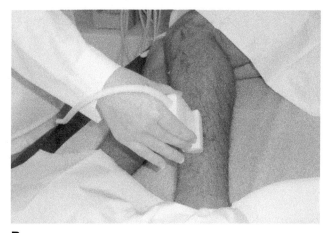

B

FIGURE i.12   Anterior approach of the left leg in transverse (A) and lateral approach of the leg in longitudinal (B).

Transducer Orientation and Interpretation

Changing the approach to view internal structures with ultrasound will have an impact on how the structure is displayed and therefore what you would actually measure. It will also affect the relative position of structures from each other, a very important concept in vascular sonography where veins, arteries, nerves, and the lymphatic system are often intimately linked. The following are some illustrations. The most important point is that it may affect your report, diagnosis, and possibly prognosis (as we will discuss in the next section on pathology of aneurysm).

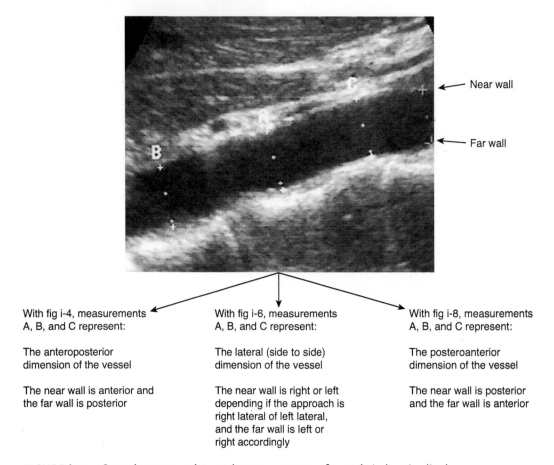

With fig i-4, measurements
A, B, and C represent:

The anteroposterior
dimension of the vessel

The near wall is anterior and
the far wall is posterior

With fig i-6, measurements
A, B, and C represent:

The lateral (side to side)
dimension of the vessel

The near wall is right or left
depending if the approach is
right lateral of left lateral,
and the far wall is left or
right accordingly

With fig i-8, measurements
A, B, and C represent:

The posteroanterior
dimension of the vessel

The near wall is posterior
and the far wall is anterior

FIGURE i.13   Scanning approaches and measurements of vessels in longitudinal.

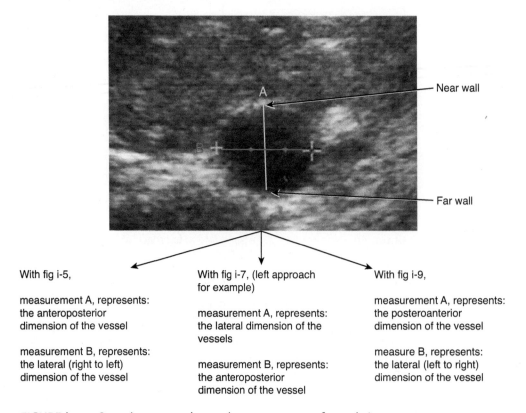

With fig i-5,

measurement A, represents:
the anteroposterior
dimension of the vessel

measurement B, represents:
the lateral (right to left)
dimension of the vessel

With fig i-7, (left approach
for example)

measurement A, represents:
the lateral dimension of the
vessels

measurement B, represents:
the anteroposterior
dimension of the vessel

With fig i-9,

measurement A, represents:
the posteroanterior
dimension of the vessel

measure B, represents:
the lateral (left to right)
dimension of the vessel

FIGURE i.14   Scanning approaches and measurements of vessels in transverse.

Anterior Approach Longitudinal

Posterior Approach Longitudinal

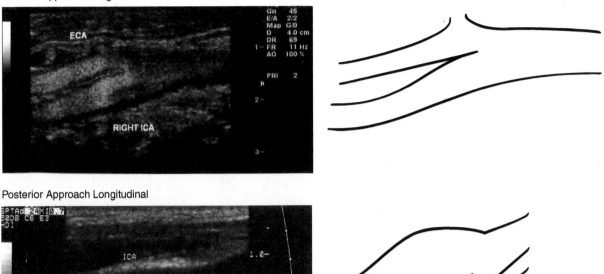

FIGURE i.15   Relative position of the ICA and ECA depending on scanning approach.

Right Side Transverse

Left Side Transverse

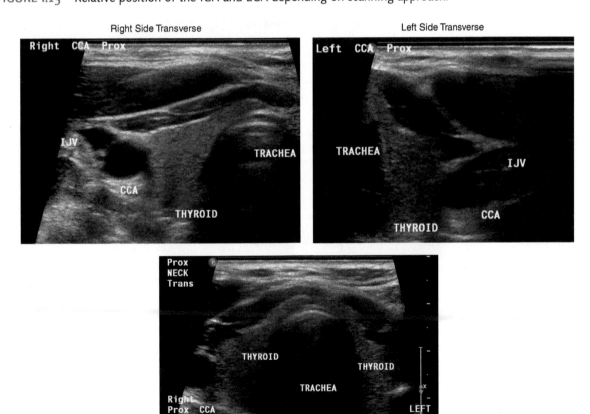

FIGURE i.16   Relative position of the ICA and ECA and anatomic variants.

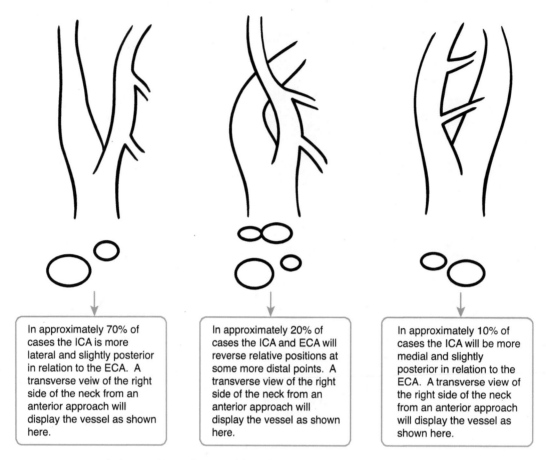

In approximately 70% of cases the ICA is more lateral and slightly posterior in relation to the ECA. A transverse veiw of the right side of the neck from an anterior approach will display the vessel as shown here.

In approximately 20% of cases the ICA and ECA will reverse relative positions at some more distal points. A transverse view of the right side of the neck from an anterior approach will display the vessel as shown here.

In approximately 10% of cases the ICA will be more medial and slightly posterior in relation to the ECA. A transverse view of the right side of the neck from an anterior approach will display the vessel as shown here.

FIGURE i.17 Relative position of a vessel (CCA) and surrounding structure (thyroid) from one side to the other.

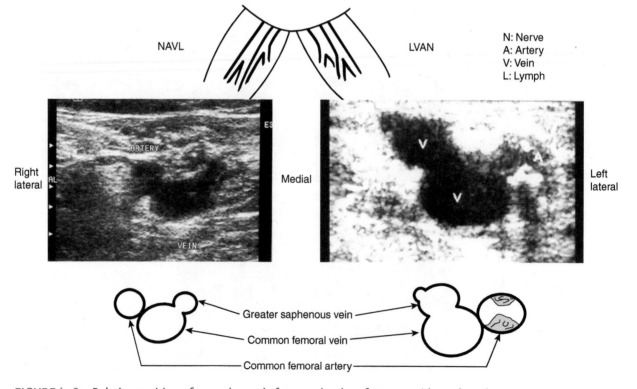

NAVL   LVAN   N: Nerve
A: Artery
V: Vein
L: Lymph

Right lateral   Medial   Left lateral

Greater saphenous vein
Common femoral vein
Common femoral artery

FIGURE i.18 Relative position of several vessels from each other, from one side to the other.

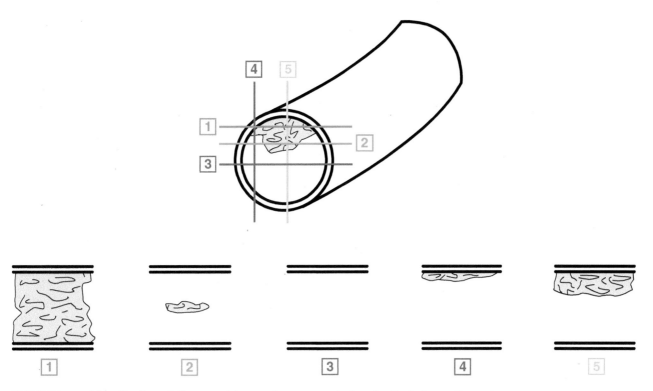

FIGURE i.19   Visualization of disease with scanning approach; longitudinal views of vessels.

Vascular Pathology Today

The following section is not intended to cover all pathologic processes known to humans as of today; rather, its main goal is to offer a sort of demystification of disease processes with the present state of knowledge in medicine. All facts are based on published data.

On Arterial Diseases

On Atherosclerosis

- Atherosclerosis is one of three major forms of arteriosclerosis or degenerative arteriopathy. The other two have been classified as medial calcific sclerosis (such as Monckeberg's) and arteriolosclerosis (involving arterioles).
- Atherosclerosis is mostly a disease process of large and medium-size arteries and their branches.
- The process also seems to be a relatively "normal" or expected degenerative process linked to aging (although the process has been noted and labeled as accelerated in some cases, without a clear understanding of the cause; the most extreme cases of accelerated atherosclerosis are seen in progeria, a genetic defect inducing a rapid aging of children).
- The precise causal relationship of environmental or lifestyle factors in the development or incidence of atherosclerosis is still not known.

- Even when strong correlations between identified risk factors and diseases have been shown, most of the underlying pathologic processes are still not fully understood.
- Most recent research tends to point to a multifactorial etiology of atherosclerosis, particularly where hemodynamic stress factors could be the primer for other factors to trigger the changes observed.
- Chronic inflammatory diseases are thought to be associated with increased arterial stiffness from probable medial calcification and in absence of atherosclerosis.
- There appears to be some regional selectivity in atherosclerosis, with a predilection for lesions to involve the femoropopliteal segments (at the adductor canal), whereas other forms of arteriosclerosis seem to be limited to the tibial arteries (such as medial calcification) when one considers the lower extremities vasculature.
- It is hypothesized that the endothelial cells may acquire or display a regional specific phenotype. This site sensitivity also appears to be linked to genetic background, immune status, gender, and oxidative stress. The role of the flow in this picture could be a primer for gene expression at this risk site.
- Fetal fatty streaks have been seen with maternal hypercholesterolemia.
- In atherosclerosis, the calcification process of plaque involves the intimal layer of the vessel from matrix vesicles that provide support for the mineralization.
- In Monckeberg's arteriosclerosis, the calcification process is different and involves the media. That process is independent of atherosclerosis (although both pathologies may coexist). Media calcification appears to be related to a glucose intolerance mechanism.

On Plaque Characteristics

- Echolucent plaques:
  - Have poor reflective contents
  - Have usually a high lipid and/or hemorrhagic content, which may point to a different pathologic etiology
  - Have been associated with a higher risk of rupture and therefore a higher incidence of neurologic events when located in the extracranial carotid system
  - Contain lysophosphatidic acid (LPA); this phospholipid, present in the lipid-rich echolucent plaque, has been shown to activate platelets and therefore induce thrombosis when released
  - Do not tend to be prone to bone formation or calcification
- Echogenic plaques:
  - Have highly reflective contents
  - Have a higher fibrous tissue component and much lower lipid content than echolucent plaques

- Have been shown to be more stable
- Do not have a high lipid core and/or hemorrhage
- The process of stabilization of echogenic plaques seems to partly involve an "ossification" (bone formation) process of the plaque, also reported as dystrophic calcification.

- It has been suggested that echolucent and echogenic plaques are two separate pathologic processes rather than one evolving into another (i.e., echolucent plaques evolving eventually to echogenic plaques).

On Aneurysms

- Most abdominal aortic aneurysms (AAA) do not predominantly display signs of atherosclerosis. Indeed aside from rupture, which still has a high morbidity and mortality, thrombus formation (not necessarily atherosclerosis when associated with aneurysm) from stagnant flow may be the next most serious complication.
- Etiology and prevalence may be pointing more toward family history and genetics than atherosclerosis (as often reported).
- Work on arteries of children with progeria shows severe and accelerated atherosclerotic process but no reported ectasia or aneurysm of the aorta, even though that vessel is primarily affected by a degenerative process in these cases.
- The most interesting link to acquired risk factors may be research and observation in elastin and/or collagen disorders and/or degenerative processes such as seen in chronic obstructive pulmonary disease (COPD), which could explain a slightly greater incidence in smokers.

- The etiology of rupture has also led to some interesting research and findings, such as:
  - Shear stress seems to induce vortices, which tend to be more significant in the distal portion of the aneurysm (greater in relatively straight rather than tortuous AAA) site, which may be more prone to rupture.
  - The rate of expansion per year seems to be a better predictor of rupture than the absolute initial size, and this seem to be positively linked to severity of COPD.
  - Some researchers have also noted the presence of small blisters or outpouchings on the vulnerable wall of ruptured AAA.
  - Ruptures seem to occur more often in the distal and posterior aspect of AAA, so the rate of expansion of the anteroposterior dimension, rather than an overall expansion in lateral or undisclosed dimension, may be a good or better predictor.

- The abdominal aorta has been shown to vary in size, without pathology, with gender, body size, and race; however, criteria for aneurysm are mostly based on size derived from studies on males. This may lead us to exclude some risks in females in whom the aneurysms were originally classified as "small."

On Buerger's Disease (Thromboangiitis Obliterans)

- Patient under the age of 35, most often with a history of heavy smoking (but not always)
- Begins at small arteries of the feet (and hands)
- Primary symptom may be intermittent claudication of the sole of the foot (often treated as foot strain because ankle pulses are still strong and palpable).
- Intolerable pain is a characteristic feature.
- Followed quickly by ulceration and gangrene (again, even with strong and palpable ankle pulses)
- The disease process inevitably progresses and ascends to the popliteal and femoral arteries (not higher).
- Fungus is almost always present in the interdigital folds.
- Disease is *always* bilateral, even though it is often more advanced in one limb compared to the other.
- Disease is sometimes preceded by patchy superficial phlebitis.
- Amputation (within 3 to 5 years of onset of disease) is unavoidable (even today!) because the course is progressive, despite periods of quiescence.
- Collateral vessels are present and have a corkscrew appearance characteristic of rapid hypertrophy and dilatation.
- Infection and sepsis of surrounding tissue often follows ulceration and gangrene and triggers edema.

On Venous Diseases

- Thrombosis:
  - The processes involved in the coagulation and lysis of thrombus are complex and interrelated.
  - Even the concepts enunciated by Virchow 150 years ago led to the consideration and/or involvement of hemodynamic (the flow of blood) and biochemical (hypercoagulability) processes.
  - Pathologies of thrombosis are mostly if not solely due to disorders of the formation or destruction of the thrombus.
  - The processes of formation and destruction of thrombus (through fibrinolysis) occur more or less at the same time. When a clot starts to form, the process of destruction is also activated.
  - There is no clear timeline to "date" the age of a thrombus in vivo. Some have proposed a 5- to 14-day period between thrombus formation and fibrinolysis (or organization of the thrombus) during an active thrombotic process.
  - Characterization of thrombus by ultrasound may be difficult, particularly when a new thrombus is superimposed on chronic changes, because the dynamic range of thrombi of different ages is very low.

- There appears to be a particular anatomic distribution, also linked to etiology, of thrombosis in the lower extremity:
  - The incidence increases from proximal to distal segments, with the peroneal veins being predominantly affected.
  - When in the proximal segment, the left side appears to be more often affected than the right (due to the anatomic position of the IVC and aorta, the left common iliac vein is often partly compressed by the right common iliac artery).
  - Thromboses arising after surgical procedures are often more prevalent at the calf level or distal segments, compared with those arising from underlying malignancy, which more likely affect proximal segments like the iliac or femoral veins.

- Varices:
  - The incidence of varicose veins is most often reported as approximately 20% of the population in the Western World.
  - The most favored theory for development of varices in the lower extremities within the last decade points to disruption of smooth muscle layers within the vein walls, leading to distension of the vein under normal pressure with a resulting valvular incompetence from spreading of valve cusps.

- Thrombosis in upper extremities:
  - The most common and increasing cause of thrombosis of upper extremity veins, including the internal jugular vein, is the presence of indwelling central catheters or pacemaker wires.
  - These causes are followed (in no particular order of importance) by rarer or unforeseen causes, such as trauma, history of hypercoagulable states, or extrinsic compression from such conditions as thoracic outlet syndrome and cancer.

On Therapies and Interventions

- Although in regard to diagnosis in the vascular laboratory, the true underlying cause or etiology for the pathologic disorder is not necessarily crucial, it becomes essential (or should) for therapy, treatment, and/or intervention.
- For example, recognizing patterns of medial calcification at the level of the tibial vessels in diabetic patients is important because these vessels will be extremely friable and suturing a bypass graft may be impossible.
- Understanding that the popliteal vein and aorta seem to respond in a similar fashion for susceptibility for aneurysms may prompt the technologist to investigate the popliteal fossae when an abdominal aneurysm is diagnosed.
- Distinguishing Buerger's disease (where there is usually no inflow problem but irreversible progression of inflammatory process of small digital arteries), for example, from other potential forms of arteriopathies (such as medial calcification with superimposed atherosclerosis in diabetes)

can guide the treating physician toward palliative care for the former and attempt of more aggressive therapies for the latter.

- Awareness and consideration of hypercoagulability and other important underlying factors, such as cancer, for thrombosis may lead to finding unsuspected causes for observed symptoms or ultrasound results.

It would be impossible to list all interventions, treatments, or therapies available, practiced, or favored. The main point raised here is that diagnostic imaging is only as good as what will be done with the results obtained. Our role as technologists is to work very closely and thus have very open communication with the referring and treating physician or health care team, so that what we can offer and obtain by the tests we perform will be meaningful for the patient. In that effort, although it is beyond the scope of our profession to offer diagnosis, we should still stay current on fundamental research in pathology. What isolated research can provide is a way for us to find an application for obtaining diagnostic information via our tests.

To conclude, at a minimum, I strongly encourage everyone to survey publications from the Cochrane Collaboration. This organization provides reviews of the recently published literature on numerous topics, which in turn offer information for developing or updating criteria, algorithms for testing, treatment plans, and so on. The website is: http://www.cochrane.org.

References and Bibliography

duPre, A. (2005). *Communicating about health: Current issues and perspectives* (2nd Ed.). New York: McGraw-Hill

Le Porrier, H. (2004). *Le medecin de Cordoue*. Paris: Seuil.

Lyons, A.S., & Petrucelli, R.J. (1987). Medicine: *An illustrated history*. New York: Harry N. Abrams, Inc.

Arterial

Anderson, J., Popovic, D., & Leers, S.A. (1992). Ergotamine-induced arterial vasospasm of the lower extremities: Diagnosis by noninvasive testing: Case study and review of the literature. *The Journal of Vascular Technology, 16,* 189–191.

Dahnjil, S., Ramaswami, G., Tegos, T., Nicolaides, A.N., Al Kutoubi, A., Lewis, J., et al. (1999). The natural history of non-calcified plaque after percutaneous transluminal angioplasty using color duplex ultrasound. *The Journal of Vascular Technology, 23,* 173–179.

Farzaneh-Far, A., Proudfoot, D., Shanahan, C., & Weissberg, P.L. (2001). Vascular and valvular calcification: Recent advances. *Heart, 85,* 13–17.

Giachelli, C.M. (2004). Vascular calcification mechanisms. *Journal of the American Society of Nephrology, 15,* 2959–2964.

Gronholdt, M.L., Wagner, A., Wiebe, B.M., Hansen, J.U., Schroeder, T.V., Wilhjelm, J.E., et al. (2001). Spiral computed tomographic imaging related to computerized ultrasonographic images of carotid plaque morphology and histology. *Journal of Ultrasound in Medicine, 20,* 451–458.

Haimovici, H. (1967). Patterns of arteriosclerotic lesions of the lower extremity. *Archives of Surgery, 95,* 918–933.

Hunt, J.L., Fairman, R., Mitchell, M.E., Carpenter, J.P., Golden, M., Khalapyan, T., et al. (2002). Bone formation in carotid plaques: A clinicopathological study. *Stroke, 33,* 1214–1219.

Marren, J.M., & Green, R.M. (1986). Doppler signal analysis in thromboangiitis obliterans: A case study. *Bruit, 10,* 177–181.

Ridker, P.M., Stampfer, M.J., & Rifai, N. (2001). Novel risk factors for systemic atherosclerosis. *The Journal of the American Medical Association, 285,* 2481–2485.

Roman, M.J., Devereaux, R.B., Schwartz, J.E., Lockshin, M.D., Paget, S.A., Davis, A., et al. (2005). Arterial stiffness in chronic inflammatory diseases. *Hypertension, 46,* 194–199.

Schwartz, C.J., Valente, A.J., & Sprague, E.A. (1993). A modern view of atherogenesis. *American Journal of Cardiology, 71,* 9B–14B.

Stehbens, W.E., Delahunt, B., Shozawa, T., & Gilbert-Barness, E. (2001). Smooth muscle cell depletion and collagen types in progeric arteries. *Cardiovascular Pathology, 10,* 131–136.

Steinman, D.A., Vorp, D.A., & Ethier, C.R. (2003). Computational modeling of arterial biomechanics: Insights into pathogenesis and treatment of vascular disease. *Journal of Vascular Surgery, 37,* 1118–1128.

VanderLaan, P.A., Reardon, C.A., & Getz, G.S. (2004). Site specificity of atherosclerosis: Site-selective responses to atherosclerotic modulators. *Arteriosclerosis, Thrombosis, and Vascular Biology, 24,* 12–22.

Vermilion, B.D. (1986). Clinical effects of diabetes mellitus on the arterial system. *Bruit, 10,* 187–191.

Walsh, D.B., Powell, R.J., Stuket, T.A., Henderson, E.L., & Cronenwelt, J.L. (1997). Superficial artery stenosis: Characteristics of progressing lesions. *Journal of Vascular Surgery, 25,* 512–521.

Wolffe, J.B., Barker, N.W., Corcoran, A.C., Duff, G.L., & Sprague, H.B. (1955). Report of committee on nomenclature of the American Society for the Study of Arteriosclerosis: Tentative classification of arteriopathies. *Circulation, 12,* 1065–1067.

Aneurysm

Barnes, S.E., & Weinberg, P.D. (1998). Contrasting patterns of spontaneous aortic disease in young and old rabbits. *Arteriosclerosis, Thrombosis, and Vascular Biology, 18,* 300–308.

Bortolotto, L.A., Hanon, O., Franconi, G., Boutouyrie, P, Legrain, S., & Girerd, X. (1999). The aging process modifies the distensibility of elastic but not muscular arteries. *Hypertension, 34,* 889–892.

Chang, J.B., Stein, T.A., Liu, J.P., & Dunn, M.E. (1997). Risk factors associated with rapid growth of small abdominal aortic aneurysms. *Surgery, 121,* 117–122.

Cronenwett, J.L., Murphy, T.F., Zelenock, G.B., Whitehouse, W.M., Jr., Lindenauer, S.M., Graham, L.M., et al. (1985). Actuarial analysis of variables associated with rupture of small abdominal aortic aneurysms. *Surgery, 98*, 472–483.

Debasso, R., Astrand, H., Bjarnegard, N., Ahlgren, A.R., Sandgren, T., & Lanne, T. (2004). The popliteal artery, an unusual muscular artery with wall properties similar to the aorta: Implications for susceptibility to aneurysm formation? *Journal of Vascular Surgery, 39*, 836–842.

Faggioli, G.L., Stella, A., Gargiulo, M., Tarantini, S., D'Addato, M., & Ricotta, J.J. (1994). Morphology of small aneurysms: Definition and impact on risk of rupture. *The American Journal of Surgery, 168*, 131–135.

Fillinger, M.F., Racusin, J., Baker, R.K., Cronenwett, J.L., Teutelink, A., Schermerhorn, M.L., et al. (2004). Anatomic characteristics of ruptured abdominal aortic aneurysm on conventional CT scans: Implications for rupture. *Journal of Vascular Surgery, 39*, 1243–1252.

Grimm, J.J., Wise, M.M., Meissner, M.H., & Nicholls, S.C. (2007). The incidence of popliteal artery aneurysms in patients with abdominal aortic aneurysms. *The Journal for Vascular Ultrasound, 31*, 71–73.

Grimshaw, G.M., & Thompson, J.M. (1997). Changes in diameter of the abdominal aorta with age: An epidemiological study. *Journal of Clinical Ultrasound, 25*, 7–13.

Lederle, F.A., Johnson, G.R., Wilson, S.E., Gordon, I.L., Chute, E.P., Littooy, F.N., et al. (1997). Relationship of age, gender, race, and body size to infrarenal aortic diameter. *Journal of Vascular Surgery, 26*, 597–601.

Multicentre Aneurysm Screening Study Group (2002). The Multicentre Aneurysm Screening Study (MASS) into the effect of abdominal aortic aneurysm screening on mortality in men: a randomized controlled trial. *The Lancet, 360*, 1531–1539.

Powell, J.T., & Greenhalgh, R.M. (2003). Small abdominal aortic aneurysms. *New England Journal of Medicine, 348*, 1895–1901.

Ricci, M.A., Kleeman, M., Case, T., & Pilcher, D.B. (1995). Normal aortic diameter by ultrasound. *The Journal of Vascular Technology, 19*, 17–19.

Sakalihasan, S., Limet, R., & Defawe, O.D. (2005). Abdominal aortic aneurysm. *The Lancet, 365*, 1577–1589.

Wills, A., Thompson, M.M., Crowther, M., Sayers, R.D., & Bell, P.R.F. (1996). Pathogenesis of abdominal aortic aneurysms: Cellular and biochemical mechanisms. *European Journal of Vascular and Endovascular Surgery, 12*, 391–400.

Venous

Anand, M., Rajagopal, K., & Rajagopal, K.R. (2005). A model for the formation and lysis of blood clots. *Pathophysiology of Haemostasis and Thrombosis, 34*, 109–120.

Gaitini, D., Beck-Razi, N., Haim, N., & Brenner, B. (2006). Prevalence of upper extremity deep venous thrombosis diagnosed by color Doppler duplex sonography in cancer patients with central venous catheters. *Journal of Ultrasound in Medicine, 25*, 1297–1303.

Heim, S.W., Schectman, J.M., Siadaty, M.S., & Philbrick, J.T. (2004). D-dimer testing for deep venous thrombosis: A metaanalysis. *Clinical Chemistry, 50,* 1136–1147.

Longley, D.G., Finlay, D.E., & Letourneau, J.G. (1993). Sonography of the upper extremity and jugular veins. *American Journal of Roentgenology, 160,* 957–962.

O'Shaughnessy, A.M., & Fitzgerald, D.E. (2001). Underlying factors influencing the development of the post-thrombotic limb. *Journal of Vascular Surgery, 34,* 247–253.

Ouriel, K., Green, R.M., Greenberg, R.K., & Clair, D.G. (2000). The anatomy of deep venous thrombosis of the lower extremity. *Journal of Vascular Surgery, 31,* 895–900.

Rubin, J.M., Xie, H., Kim, K., Weitzel, W.F., Emelianov, S.Y., Aglyamov, S.R., et al. (2006). Sonographic elasticity imaging of acute and chronic deep venous thrombosis in humans. *Journal of Ultrasound in Medicine, 25,* 1179–1186.

Travers, J.P., Brookes, C.E., Evans, J., Baker, D.M., Kent, C., Makin, G.S., et al. (1996). Assessment of wall structure and composition of varicose veins with reference to collagen, elastin and smooth muscle content. *European Journal of Vascular and Endovascular Surgery, 11,* 230–237.

Wakai, A., Gleeson, A., & Winter, D. (2003). Role of fibrin D-dimer testing in emergency medicine. *Emergency Medicine Journal, 20,* 319–325.

Contents

CHAPTER

1

PART I: HEAD AND NECK

Testing the Intracranial Circulation

Chapter Outline

Vessels

Structures

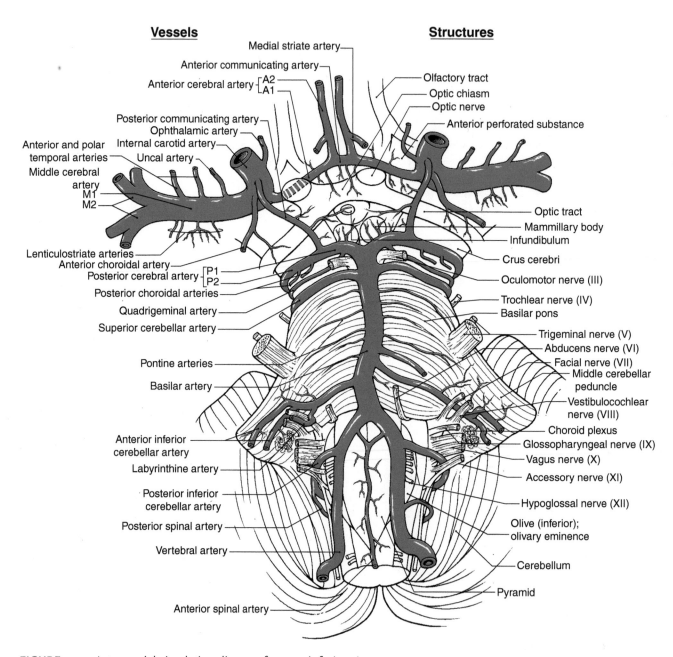

Medial striate artery

Anterior communicating artery

Anterior cerebral artery ⎡A2
                        ⎣A1

Posterior communicating artery

Ophthalmic artery

Internal carotid artery

Anterior and polar temporal arteries

Uncal artery

Middle cerebral artery
M1
M2

Lenticulostriate arteries

Anterior choroidal artery

Posterior cerebral artery ⎡P1
                         ⎣P2

Posterior choroidal arteries

Quadrigeminal artery

Superior cerebellar artery

Pontine arteries

Basilar artery

Anterior inferior cerebellar artery

Labyrinthine artery

Posterior inferior cerebellar artery

Posterior spinal artery

Vertebral artery

Anterior spinal artery

Olfactory tract

Optic chiasm

Optic nerve

Anterior perforated substance

Optic tract

Mammillary body

Infundibulum

Crus cerebri

Oculomotor nerve (III)

Trochlear nerve (IV)

Basilar pons

Trigeminal nerve (V)

Abducens nerve (VI)

Facial nerve (VII)

Middle cerebellar peduncle

Vestibulocochlear nerve (VIII)

Choroid plexus

Glossopharyngeal nerve (IX)

Vagus nerve (X)

Accessory nerve (XI)

Hypoglossal nerve (XII)

Olive (inferior); olivary eminence

Cerebellum

Pyramid

FIGURE 1.1.   Intracranial circulation diagram from an inferior view.

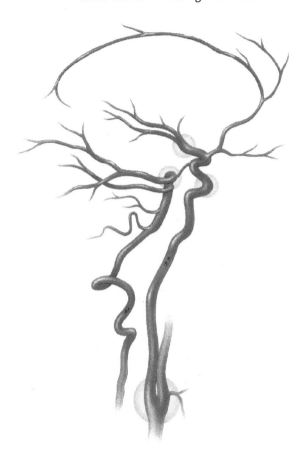

FIGURE 1.2.   Highlighted areas represent common sites of stenosis.

General Concepts in Intracranial Circulation

Across the United States of America, the evaluation of the intracranial arteries by Doppler alone or duplex ultrasound is usually not part of the routine spectrum of tests available. Although all registered vascular technologists possess at least theoretical exposure to transcranial vascular tests (it is a required topic for the ARDMS exam), many do not have the opportunities to practice the skills regularly.

Reasons for such trends may depend on the patient population serviced by the vascular lab (for example, centers caring for population with sickle cell anemia), as well as be based on the medical or surgical services available (for example, centers with large neurologic units or trauma services).

However, with an increased demand for noninvasive and safer imaging techniques, as well as an aging population, we cannot discount the role intracranial or transcranial testing by Doppler or duplex ultrasound may play in the future.

The following sections will offer an overview of the techniques, normal findings and pathologies.

■ Examination of the intracranial arteries must respond to specific questions which could be answered by the results obtained.

■ Using transcranial testing by Doppler or duplex ultrasound to look at sites of embolic or ischemic stroke may not yield as valuable information as other tests could.

■ The main uses for transcranial testing by Doppler or duplex ultrasound are at this point focused on the following indications:
  • Evaluation of pathologies associated with sickle cell anemia
  • Detection of aneurysms
  • Detection of arteriovenous fistulae or other malformations
  • Monitoring vasospasm after intracranial aneurysm repair
  • Monitoring embolus formation during carotid endarterectomy and/or stenting of extracranial carotid arteries

■ Other uses of transcranial testing by Doppler or duplex ultrasound may be:
  • Evaluation of brain death. Although this can be achieved by evaluating the extracranial carotid and vertebral arteries where all arteries would display highly resistive flow bilaterally. These results should be interpreted with caution, as they can lead to false positive.
  • Evaluation of collateral flow in case of severe stenosis, occlusion, or agenesis of extracranial or intracranial vessels, or completeness of the circle of Willis. However this could probably be achieved with better specificity and sensitivity with other medical imaging techniques.

Tips/Rationale

■ Prepare the instrument correctly and DO NOT change the setting for the direction of flow at any point during the exam. As will be emphasized later, the direction of flow, particularly with Doppler, provides most of your identification and diagnostic criteria.

■ Have a realistic outlook for images.
  • A patient with sickle cell anemia will likely image well due to their young age and small cranial dimensions.
  • A patient with possible aneurysm will usually be older, have a large skull, and may have temporal window limitations due to ossification, resulting in lower quality imaging and color fill.
  • In a patient who suffered a head trauma and resulting subdural hematoma, there may be a midline shift of internal vessels (in relation to the depth you may normally use to access the vessel) on the side of the hematoma.
  • Use gain, color scale, and color-write priority adjustments, color persistence settings, and even low-flow settings, if available, for color image optimization.

- Keep the goals of the study in mind for each type of patient.
  - For a patient with sickle cell anemia, the goal is primarily Doppler velocities within the vessels; the secondary goal is imaging.
  - For a patient with potential aneurysm, the goal is primarily detailed imaging of location.
  - In a patient evaluation post-op aneurysm intervention, the goals are again primarily Doppler velocities to detect vasospasm and flow in general and, secondarily, detailed imaging of the (hopefully nonfilling) aneurysmal sac.
- Be very familiar with the intracranial vascular anatomy and relationships of vessels to landmarks visible to ultrasound. "Keep this book handy for reference during the exam!"
  - Via the temporal window, look for the shallow "V"-shaped, echogenic bony protrusion of the "sphenoid process," medial to the confluence of the anterior cerebral, carotid siphon, and posterior communicating arteries.
  - Via the foramen magnum window, follow the vertebral arteries to the basilar artery, noting the left and right branches of the posterior cerebral arteries.
  - Via the transorbital window, use the back of the orbit and the ophthalmic artery to orient to the anterior communicating, anterior cerebral, and middle cerebral arteries.
- Be sure of your image orientation!
  - Keep in mind that venous flow intracranially may display marked pulsatility.
  - Be sure of your vessel by asking "Which direction should this flow be going?" and relating the answer to the transducer orientation and positioning.
- Know what the Doppler waveforms should look like for each major vessel, including characteristics and direction. "Keep this book handy for reference during the exam!"
- Pay attention to power exposure indexes in relation to the patient!
  - Use of some presets without adjustment of output settings may result in high mechanical index (MI) and thermal index for soft tissue (TIS) exposures. Although still likely to be safe, there is no reason to expose a sickle cell infant or toddler to high power levels needlessly.
  - Adjust power output down and use gain settings.

Protocol Algorithm

Baseline exam as described in the test sequence in the following section. Review indications and history

Particular attention to ICA and MCA segments, for:
- Ischemic stroke due to stenosis (10% of all stroke)
- Establishing baseline and following vasospasm
- Sickle cell anemia evaluation

Particular attention to vertebral/basilar segments, for:
- Ischemic stroke in the posterior circulation, to evaluate stenosis/occlusion
- Collateralization due to occlusion of other vessels and/or anatomical variants

Particular attention to ophthalmic artery for:
- Collateralization of flow

FIGURE 1.3.   Protocol algorithm.

Doppler Exam and Duplex Exam of the Intracranial Circulation

Test Preparation

Keep your patient comfortable for each window used. Sometimes a sitting position can be better tolerated by a patient, particularly when using the foramen magnum as a window. A sitting position (for the patient) may also allow for a better positioning of the arm of the sonographer holding the transducer, in regard to the angles between the shoulder, elbow, and wrist.

Testing Sequence

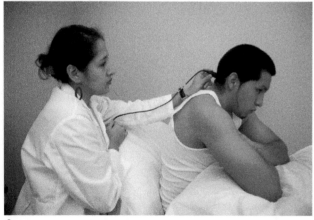
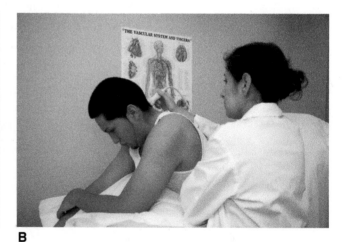

A   **B**

FIGURE 1.4.   Transducer (Doppler) placed on occipital window, patient sitting. The patient may also be supine in a right or left decubitus position to access the foramen magnum.

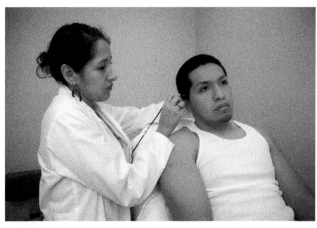

FIGURE 1.5. Transducer (Doppler) placed on right temporal window, patient sitting.

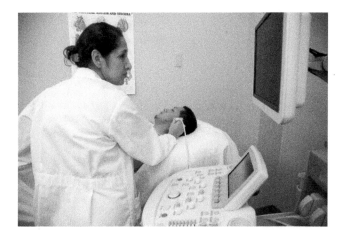

FIGURE 1.6. Transducer (duplex) placed on left temporal window, patient supine.

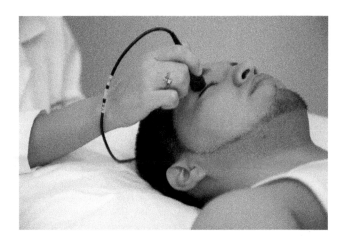

FIGURE 1.7. Transducer (Doppler) placed on orbital window, patient supine. The use of duplex for transorbital examination requires that the manufacturer received FDA approval for such application.

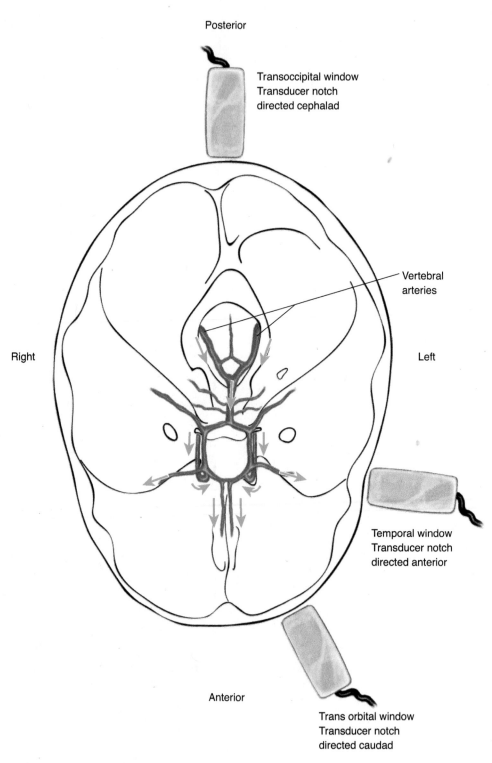

FIGURE 1.8.   Transducer position in relation to intracranial arterial circulation.

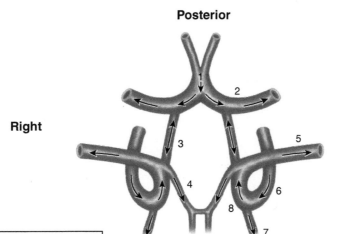

Occipital Window

Vertebral arteries: flow away

Basilar artery: flow away

Posterior

Right

Left

Intracranial Circulation

1– Basilar Artery
2– Posterior Cerebral Artery (P1: first arrow, and P2: second arrow segments)
3– Posterior Communicating Artery
4– Anterior Cerebral Artery
5– Middle Cerebral Artery
6– Internal Carotid Artery
7– Opthalmic Artery
8– Carotid Siphon
Arrow indicates direction of flow

Anterior

Temporal Window

MCA: flow toward (for ipsilateral side), flow away (for contralateral side)

ACA/MCA: Bidirectional flow (toward for MCA, and away for ACA)

ACA: flow away

PCA: P1 flow toward, P2 flow away

ICA: flow toward or away

Trans Orbital Window

Opthalmic artery: flow toward

Carotid Siphon: flow toward, bidirectional and away

FIGURE 1.9. Flow direction expected by Doppler or duplex, with transducer placed as indicated previously, for each of the main vessels of the circle of Willis.

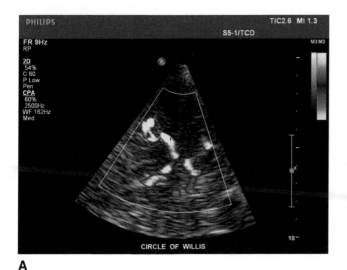

A

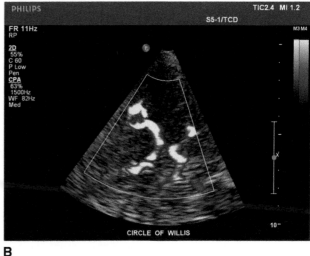

B

FIGURE 1.10. Circle of Willis by duplex ultrasound and color flow. Courtesy of Philips.

Results and Interpretation

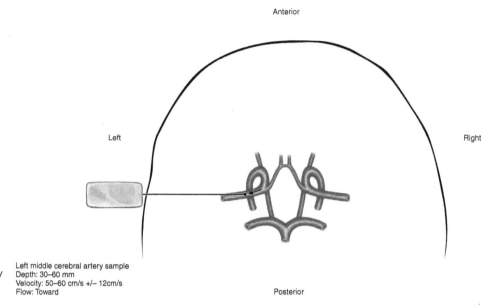

FIGURE 1.11.   Transducer's position for sampling of MCA from temporal window. The transducer is placed practically perpendicular to the body.

Left middle cerebral artery sample
Depth: 30–60 mm
Velocity: 50–60 cm/s +/– 12cm/s
Flow: Toward

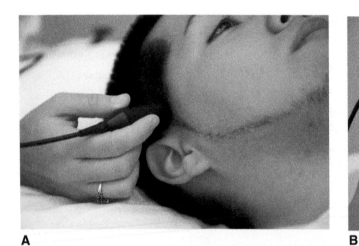

A

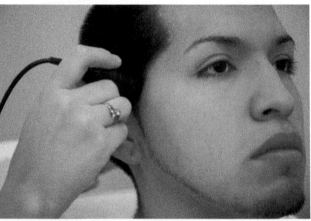

B

FIGURE 1.12.   Transducer's position for sampling of MCA from temporal window (here by Doppler for the right MCA). The transducer is placed practically perpendicular to the body.

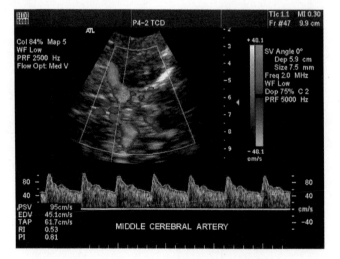

FIGURE 1.13.   Normal MCA spectral and color Doppler with duplex ultrasound.
Courtesy of Philips.

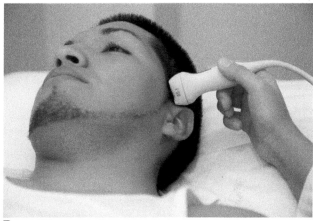

FIGURE 1.14. Left MCA/ACA bifurcation sample. D: 55-65; V: variable; F: toward for MCA, away for ACA.

Left middle cerebral/anterior cerebral bifurcation sample
Depth: 55–65 mm
Velocity: Variable
Flow: Toward (for MCA), away (for ACA)

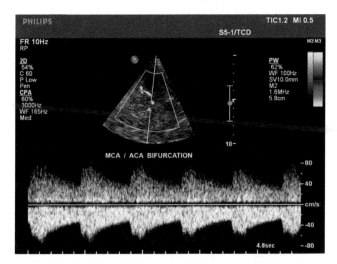

A   **B**

FIGURE 1.15. Transducer's position for sampling at the MCA/ACA from the temporal window (A: by Doppler on the right; B: by duplex on the left). The transducer's position will remain basically the same as for the MCA sampling, but the sampling will be acquired at a greater depth.

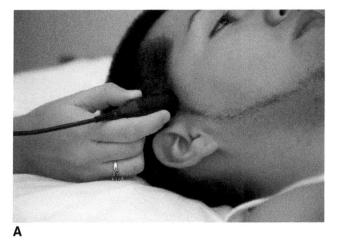

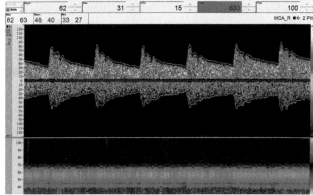

FIGURE 1.16. Normal MCA/ACA flow separation by spectral and color Doppler with duplex ultrasound. Positive flow (toward transducer) is MCA, negative flow (away from transducer) is ACA. Courtesy of Philips.

FIGURE 1.17. Normal MCA/ACA flow separation by spectral Doppler. Positive flow (toward transducer) is MCA, negative flow (away from transducer) is ACA. Courtesy of Compumedics.

Anterior

Left

Right

Left anterior cerebral artery sample
Depth: 60–80 mm
Velocity: 50 cm/s +/– 12 cm/s
Flow: Away

Posterior

FIGURE 1.18. Transducer's position for sampling ACA from temporal window. The transducer will be angled slightly more anteriorly than for MCA sampling. The sampling will also be at a greater depth.

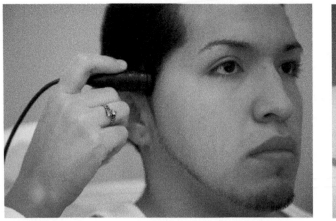

A

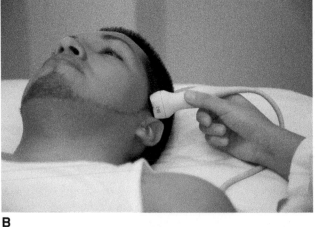

B

FIGURE 1.19. Transducer's position for sampling ACA and terminal ICA from temporal window by Doppler (A) and by duplex on the left (B).

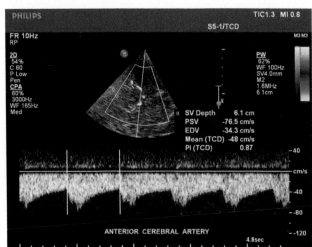

FIGURE 1.20. Normal ACA spectral and color Doppler with duplex ultrasound. Courtesy of Philips.

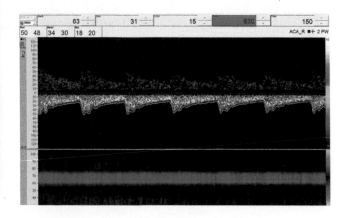

FIGURE 1.21. Normal ACA spectral Doppler. Courtesy of Compumedics.

Anterior

Left

Right

Left terminal internal carotid
artery sample
Depth: 55–65 mm
Velocity: Varies
Flow: Toward

Posterior

FIGURE 1.22.   Transducer's position for sampling the terminal ICA from temporal window. As with the ACA the transducer will be angled more anteriorly than for MCA sampling, but the depth for sampling will be similar to MCA/ACA sampling.

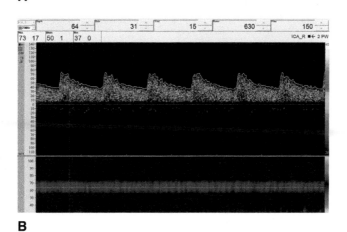

A

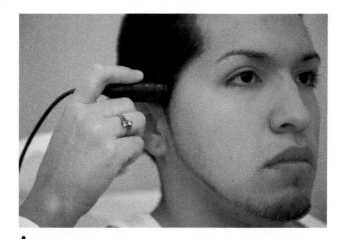

B

FIGURE 1.23.   Normal terminal ICA waveforms. Courtesy of Compumedics.

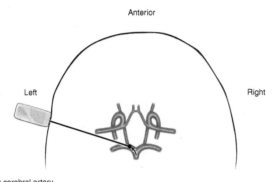

Left

Right

Anterior

Posterior

Left posterior cerebral artery
(P1) sample
Depth: 60–75 mm
Velocity: 39–42 cm/s +/– 10 cm/s
Flow: Toward

FIGURE 1.24. Transducer's position for sampling PCA, P1 segment, from temporal window. The transducer will be angled posteriorly and the sampling acquired at a slightly greater depth than P2 segment.

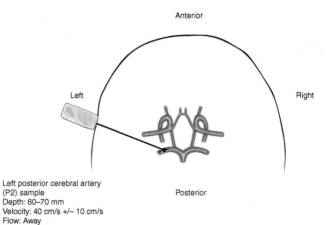

Left

Right

Anterior

Posterior

Left posterior cerebral artery
(P2) sample
Depth: 60–70 mm
Velocity: 40 cm/s +/– 10 cm/s
Flow: Away

FIGURE 1.25. Transducer's position for sampling PCA, P2 segment, from temporal window. The transducer will be angled posteriorly and the sampling acquired at a slightly lower depth than P1 segment. The direction of flow on the spectrum will distinguish the segment: toward the transducer for P1 and away from the transducer for P2.

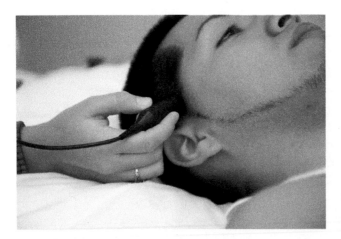

FIGURE 1.26. Transducer's position for sampling PCA segments from temporal window, here by Doppler on the right.

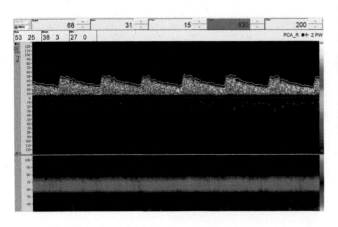

FIGURE 1.27. Normal PCA, P1 segment, spectral Doppler. Courtesy of Compumedics.

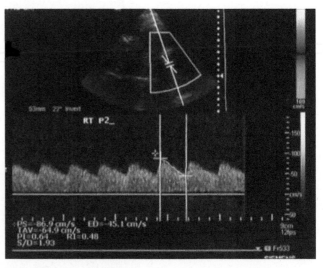

FIGURE 1.28. Slightly abnormal PCA, P2 segment, spectral Doppler in a patient with sickle cell anemia. Note: Even though the spectral flow is appearing above the baseline (the spectrum was manually inverted), the flow is away from the transducer (the peak systolic velocity is recorded as: −87 cm/s).

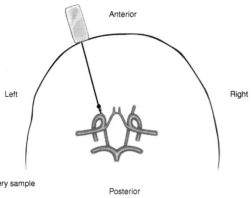

Left opthalmic artery sample
Depth: 40–60 mm
Velocity: 20 cm/s +/– 5 cm/s
Flow: Toward

FIGURE 1.29. Transducer's position for sampling ophthalmic artery from orbital window. The transducer is placed on a closed eyelid (make sure to ask the patient to remove contact lenses and inquire about any existing conditions contraindicated for the study, such as recent eye surgery or infection). The sampling is placed at a rather shallow depth.

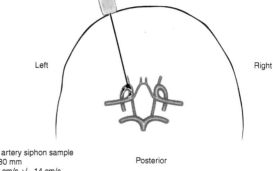

Left carotid artery siphon sample
Depth: 60–80 mm
Velocity: 47 cm/s +/– 14 cm/s
Flow: Away, bidirectional, toward

FIGURE 1.30. Transducer's position for sampling carotid siphon from orbital window. The transducer is placed in the same fashion and with the same recommendations as for the ophthalmic artery but the sampling is placed at a greater depth.

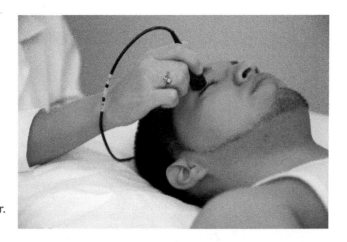

FIGURE 1.31. Normal ophthalmic artery spectral Doppler. Courtesy of Compumedics.

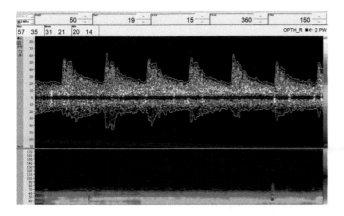

FIGURE 1.32. Transducer's position for sampling ophthalmic artery and carotid siphon from orbital window, here by Doppler on right. Note: Caution should be exercised in using this window with duplex ultrasound by checking with the ultrasound manufacturer.

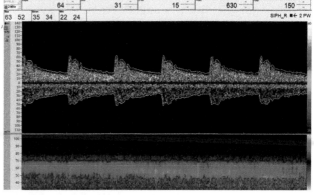

FIGURE 1.33. Normal carotid siphon spectral Doppler. Courtesy of Compumedics.

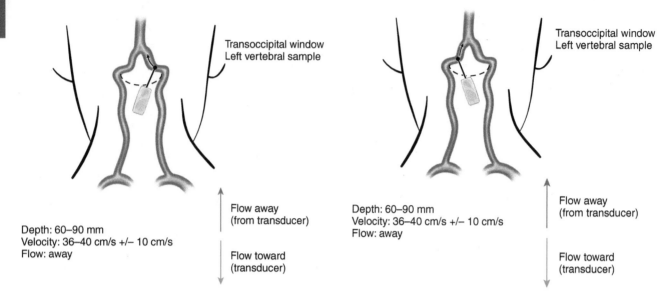

Transoccipital window
Left vertebral sample

Depth: 60–90 mm
Velocity: 36–40 cm/s +/– 10 cm/s
Flow: away

Flow away
(from transducer)

Flow toward
(transducer)

Transoccipital window
Left vertebral sample

Depth: 60–90 mm
Velocity: 36–40 cm/s +/– 10 cm/s
Flow: away

Flow away
(from transducer)

Flow toward
(transducer)

FIGURE 1.34. Transducer's position for sampling the right vertebral arteries. The transducer will be angled superiorly and rotated slightly to either side for sampling each vertebral artery.

FIGURE 1.35. Transducer's position for sampling the left vertebral arteries The transducer will be angled superiorly and rotated slightly to either side for sampling each vertebral artery.

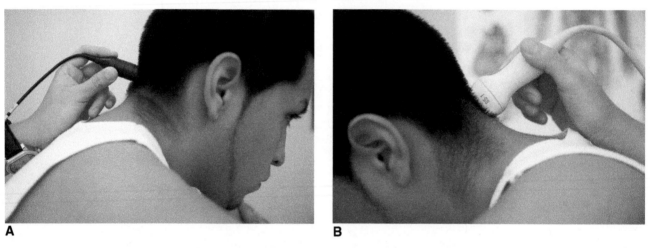

A

B

FIGURE 1.36. Transducer's position for sampling vertebral and basilar arteries from occipital window by Doppler (A) and by duplex ultrasound (B).

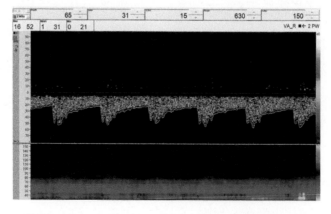

FIGURE 1.37. Normal vertebral artery spectral Doppler.
Courtesy of Compumedics.

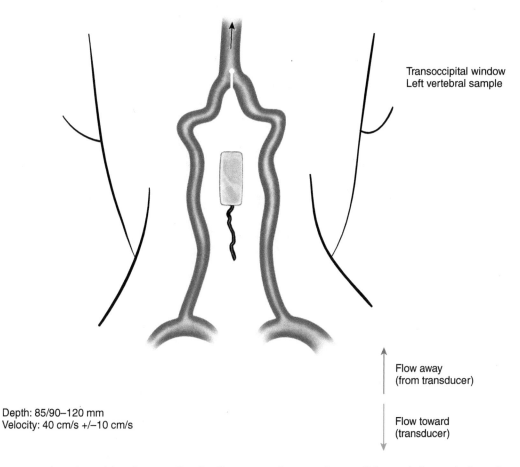

Transoccipital window
Left vertebral sample

Flow away
(from transducer)

Flow toward
(transducer)

Depth: 85/90–120 mm
Velocity: 40 cm/s +/–10 cm/s

FIGURE 1.38.   Transducer's position for sampling basilar artery. The transducer will be angled superiorly and straight at a greater depth than for vertebral arteries sampling.

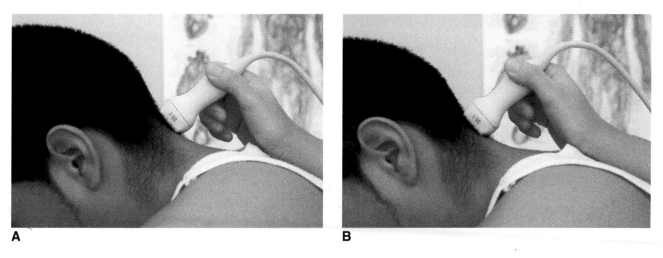

A   B

FIGURE 1.39.   Transducer's position for basilar artery.

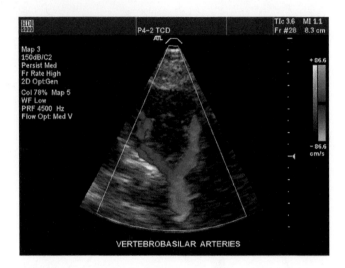

FIGURE 1.40. Normal vertebral and basilar arteries color Doppler by duplex ultrasound. Courtesy of Philips.

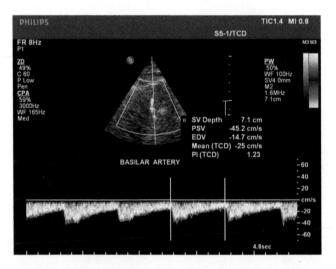

FIGURE 1.41. Normal basilar artery color and spectral Doppler by duplex ultrasound. Courtesy of Philips.

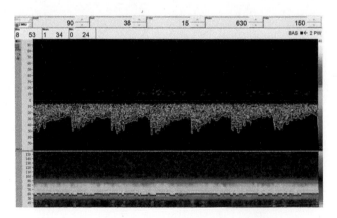

FIGURE 1.42. Normal basilar artery spectral Doppler. Courtesy of Compumedics.

TABLE 1.1: **Results and Interpretations with Pathology**

Pathology/Indication	Results	Interpretation
Stenosis	Increased velocities at the stenotic site (as compared to the same location on the contralateral side)	x2 for 50%, and x3 for 75% Poststenosis turbulence Note 1: The most reliable site for determining stenosis accurately is the MCA segment. Note 2: Remember to consider the patient's age because with increasing age, the velocities are likely to decrease as observed in the extracranial circulation; also consider the patient's medical history because, for example, anemia is likely to increase flow velocities as a result of decrease in blood viscosity.
Occlusion	No flow detected	Note: Ensure that you are actually insonating the proper vessel at the proper angle and depth.
Vasospasm	Increased velocities and documented on sequential (daily) examination	The most reliable site for detection of vasospasm is again the MCA segment. The velocities on sequential Doppler will increase to more than 120 cm/s and likely: 200 cm/s, and the MCA/ICA systolic velocity ration would be: 3.
Arteriovenous malformations or fistulae	Increased systolic and diastolic velocities with accompanied low pulsatility indices in the artery supplying the fistula; reduced flow in the adjacent arteries or segments may also be seen	This becomes relatively difficult to identify without a baseline study; however, the recommended velocities range, as expressed in the previous section, will serve as a guideline. Turbulence within the Doppler spectrum will be seen.
Sickle cell anemia	Increased velocities in the intracranial ICA and MCA	Refer to the STOP protocol found in the appendices. Velocities between 170 and 199 cm/s are suspicious, and velocities: 200 cm/s with correlated medical history represent abnormal findings.

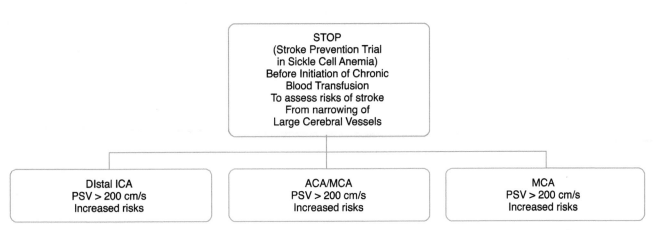

Risks of Stroke from involvement of the Vertebrobasilar (PCA segments, as well as Vertebral arteries and Basilar artery) System are rare but still exist and follow same criteria.

FIGURE 1.43.   Protocol for investigation for blood transfusion qualification of patients with sickle cell anemia.

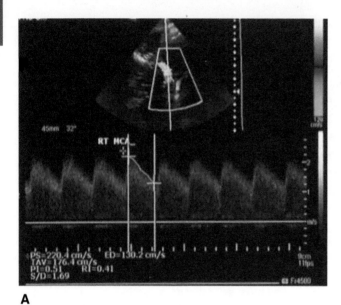

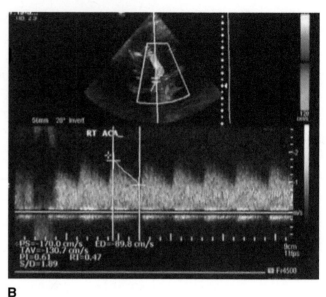

A   B

FIGURE 1.44. ACA and MCA in patient with sickle cell anemia. (A) Right MCA through right temporal window. Peak Systolic velocity: 220 cm/s; end diastolic velocity: 130 cm/s; flow direction: toward, abnormal finding (PSV : 200 cm/s). (B) Right ACA through right temporal window. Peak systolic velocity: 170 cm/s; end diastolic velocity: 89 cm/s; flow direction: away, marginal (conditional) finding (PSV ≥ 170 cm/s).

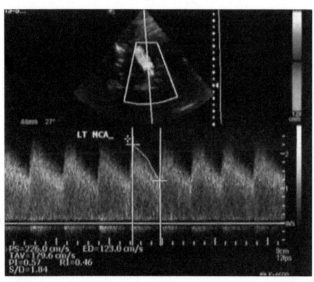

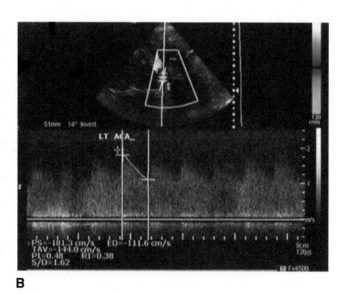

A   B

FIGURE 1.45. ACA and MCA in patient with sickle cell anemia. (A) Left MCA through left temporal window. Peak systolic velocity: 226 cm/s; end diastolic velocity: 123 cm/s; flow direction: toward, abnormal finding (PSV : 200 cm/s). (B) Left ACA through left temporal window. Peak systolic velocity: 181 cm/s; end diastolic velocity: 112 cm/s; flow direction: away, marginal (conditional) finding (PSV ≥ 170 cm/s).

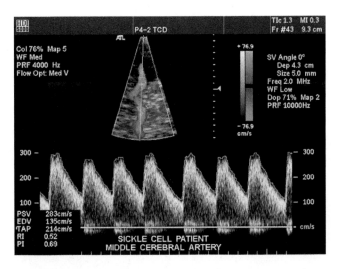

FIGURE 1.46. MCA in patient with sickle cell anemia.
Courtesy of Philips.

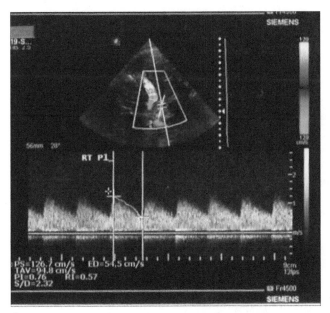

A

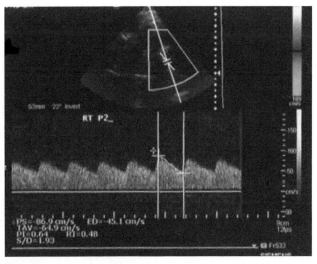

B

FIGURE 1.47. PCA (P1 and P2 segments) in patient with sickle cell anemia. (A) Right PCA (P1 segment) through right temporal window. Peak systolic velocity: 127 cm/s; end diastolic velocity: 54 cm/s; flow direction: toward. (B) Right PCA (P2 segment) through right temporal window. Peak systolic velocity: 87 cm/s; End diastolic velocity: 45 cm/s; flow direction: away.

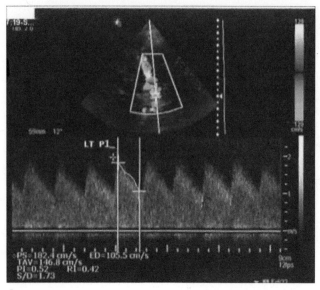
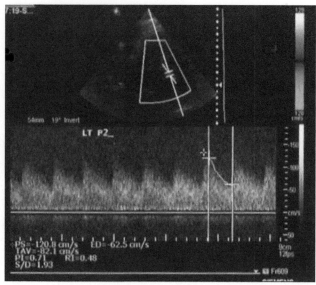

A   **B**

FIGURE 1.48.   PCA (P1 and P2 segments) in patient with sickle cell anemia. (A) Left PCA (P1 segment) through left temporal window. Peak systolic velocity: 182 cm/s; end diastolic velocity: 105 cm/s; flow direction: toward, marginal (conditional) finding (PSV ≥ 170 cm/s). (B) Left PCA (P1 segment) through left temporal window. Peak systolic velocity: 120 cm/s; end diastolic velocity: 62 cm/s; flow direction: away.

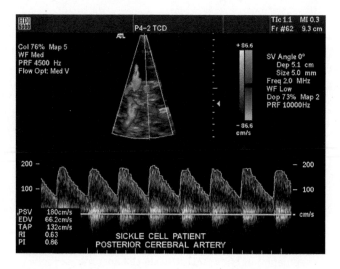

FIGURE 1.49.   PCA in patient with sickle cell anemia. Courtesy of Philips.

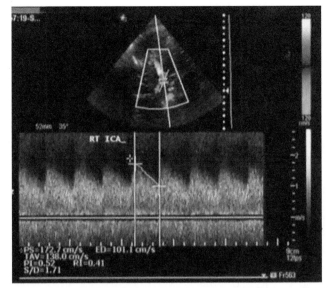

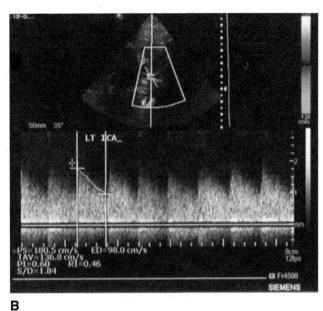

A   **B**

FIGURE 1.50.   Right and left terminal internal carotid arteries in patient with sickle cell anemia. (A) Right ICA terminal segment through right temporal window. Peak systolic velocity: 172 cm/s; end diastolic velocity: 100 cm/s; flow direction: mostly toward and bidirectional, marginal (conditional) finding (PSV ≥ 170 cm/s). (B) Left ICA terminal segment through left temporal window. Peak systolic velocity: 180 cm/s; end diastolic velocity: 98 cm/s; flow direction: mostly toward and bidirectional, marginal (conditional) finding (PSV ≥ 170 cm/s).

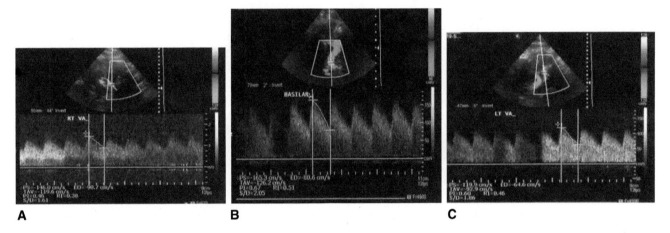

A   **B**   **C**

FIGURE 1.51.   Right and left vertebral arteries and basilar arteries in patient with sickle cell anemia. Basilar, right, and left vertebral arteries through occipital window; basilar: PSV: 165 cm/s, EDV: 80 cm/s, flow away; right vertebral: PSV: 146 cm/s, EDV: 90 cm/s, flow away; left vertebral: PSV: 120 cm/s, EDV: 65 cm/s, flow away.

Concluding Tips

- If your lab is going to offer this testing modality, get trained before starting to schedule patients for the exam. Without training, it will be a frustrating experience and thus will not help anyone, particularly the patient.

- Keep in mind that many patients CANNOT be evaluated by these methods, particularly older patients, because the skull bones are fused tightly and have ossified, which limits the available windows. In addition, the foramen magnum window involves placing the patient in a position that may be quite uncomfortable and therefore difficult to maintain for any extended period of time.

PART I: HEAD AND NECK

Testing the Extracranial Circulation

Chapter Outline

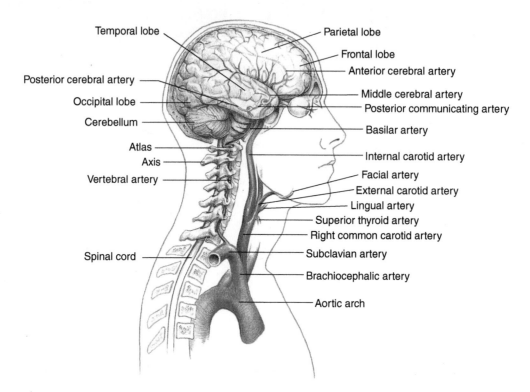

FIGURE 2.1.   Diagram of the extracranial arterial circulation.

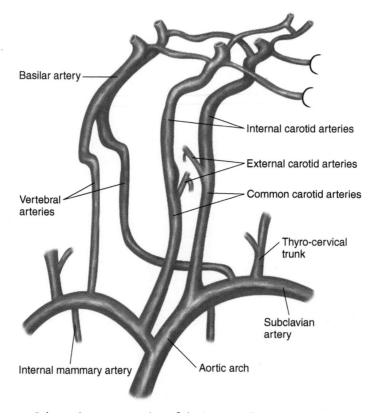

FIGURE 2.2.   Schematic representation of the intra- and extracranial arterial circulation.

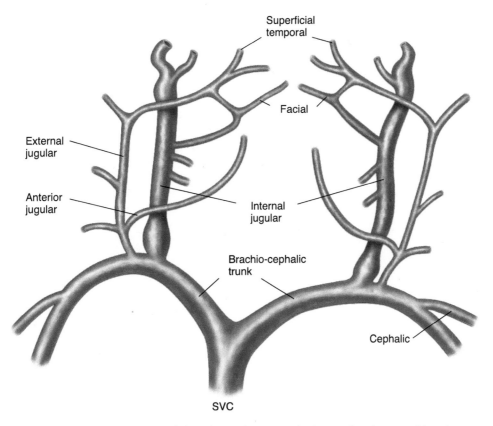

FIGURE 2.3. Schematic representation of the relation between the internal and external jugular venous system.

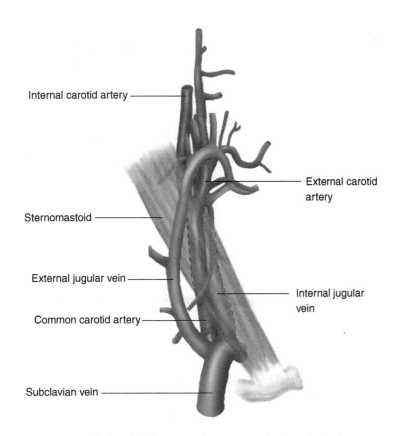

FIGURE 2.4. Relationship between the extracranial arterial and venous systems.

General Concepts in Extracranial Arterial Evaluation

The testing of the extracranial circulation by ultrasound has mainly focused on the evaluation of the carotid/vertebral arterial system. Duplex ultrasound has become a reliable modality for physicians to evaluate symptoms and their etiologies, as well as to plan treatment procedures. The extracranial venous system will be explored in the second part of this chapter.

■ A test should always be offered and performed in response to a question.

■ The question or questions could be related to diagnosis, treatment, or in some cases even prognosis.

   • On diagnosis:
      ○ Are the symptoms consistent with a neurologic deficit from a reduction or an interruption of flow to the tissue?
      ○ Could the symptoms possibly be caused by problems other than vascular?
      ○ Are the symptoms and findings consistent with the patient's age, health status, and medical history?

   • On treatment:
      ○ Are the findings amenable to available intervention?
      ○ Are there any special considerations for available interventions that need to be reported, such as anatomic variation, high bifurcation, long segment of disease, or suspicion of more intracranial problems?

   • On prognosis:
      ○ Is the ultrasound test sufficient for planning intervention?
      ○ Are the ultrasound findings giving a complete picture?

■ Of course many of these questions will need to be answered by the physician or team of physicians handling the case, but it is part of your role as a sonographer to ensure that you provide all possible information available from the test you performed and the data you gathered during your examination, including the patient's medical history.

Tips/Rationale

■ The carotid arteries, mostly through the internal carotid artery, as well as the vertebral arteries, are the main channels for oxygen delivery to the brain.

   • These vessels can be narrowed or obstructed by atherosclerotic plaque, thrombus, or vasospasm.

   • These vessels can also be prone to other problems such as dissection or routes for emboli.

   • The symptoms associated with the pathologies mentioned vary tremendously from no observable symptoms, to focal and/or transient symptoms, to potentially extensive and/or irreversible symptoms and damages to the tissues.

- Therefore, *history is/should be a crucial component* of the exam and should focus on:
  - Symptoms: their length in time, their severity, and their apparition
  - Age of the patient: some pathologies are rare in certain age groups
  - Family: some pathologies are hereditary
- If the patient cannot answer, ask a very reliable source! Live-in family members are usually a great asset because they can give you an account of subtle or sudden changes in the patient's status.
- Although the basic protocol for examination will be the same, the history should lead you to focus on specific findings, such as the integrity of the intima; the pattern and appearance of the plaque; the pattern, direction, and velocity of the flow; the characteristics on the Doppler waveforms; and differential diagnosis.

Protocol Algorithm

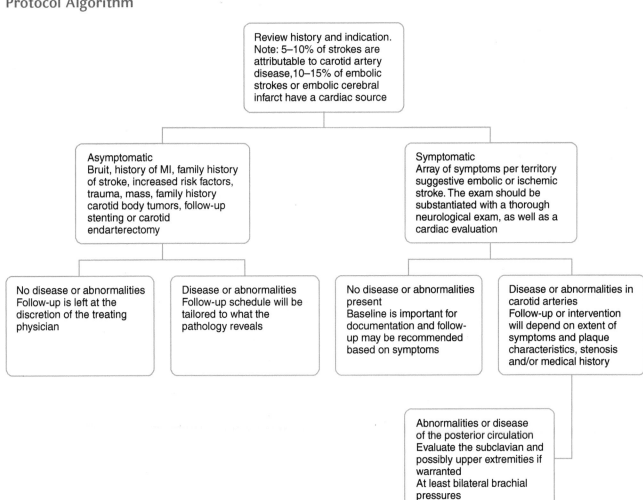

FIGURE 2.5.   Algorithm for examination.

Duplex Exam of the Extracranial Arterial Circulation

Test Preparation

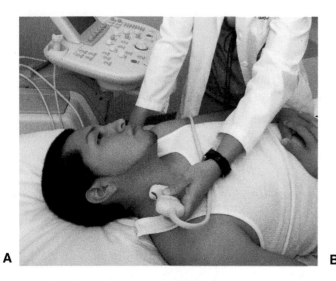

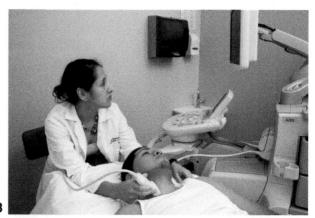

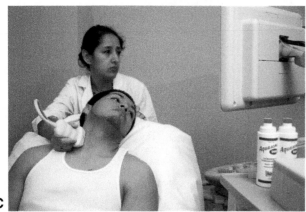

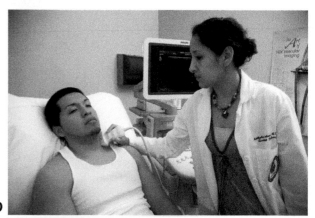

A

B

C

D

FIGURE 2.6. Examples of possible positions, of transducer and sonographer, to evaluate the vessels of the neck (carotid system, vertebral arteries and veins, jugular venous system).

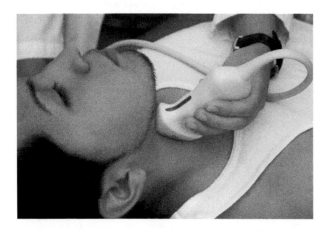

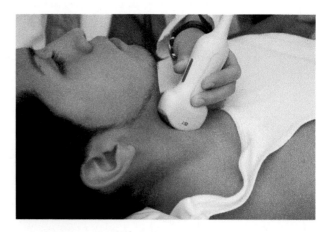

FIGURE 2.7. A linear transducer with high frequencies is typically the transducer of choice for the evaluation of the vessels of the neck.

FIGURE 2.8. A curved transducer with lower frequencies (usually used for the evaluation of the abdomen) can be used in patients with a large neck or with swelling from an indwelling catheter or recent surgical procedure, such as endarterectomy.

Testing Sequence

Note 1: There is technically no right or wrong order as to what should constitute the sequence, which is defined as the chronological order in which the images are to be taken, and therefore the approach to the exam. What is important is that all steps are documented properly, substantiating the history you gathered and emphasizing the area of suspicion (based on presenting symptoms and medical/surgical history). However, it is probably an advantage to start the exam in B mode with the transducer positioned in transverse from the base of the neck and moving distally. This approach will give you a very quick overview of the anatomy (including, but not limited to, positioning of the arteries and veins, branches, variants, tortuosity, bifurcation level, etc.), as well as an idea of the pathology you will encounter.

Note 2: The test sequence will not follow here any particular protocol. This should be tailored to your patient's population and clinical practice. However, to support the efforts of the Intersocietal Commission for the Accreditation of Vascular Laboratories (ICAVL) in providing consistency in examination across the nation, the exam will follow the recommendations of this organization in regard to the minimum and recommended additional images to obtain (available at: http://www.icavl.org/icavl/pdfs/extracranial2007.pdf).

Note 3: Always start your exam and therefore optimize your image in B mode or gray scale. Color and power Doppler are important tools in vascular ultrasound but should be used wisely and sometimes sparingly (i.e., when plaque obscures the remaining vessel lumen and the area of highest stenosis becomes difficult to visualize, or if dissection is noted); otherwise, most of the exam can be performed in gray scale with pulsed wave (PW) Doppler interrogation at specific and representative locations. Sample Protocol:

1. Sweep through the entire system, starting at the base of the neck and moving cephalad to the most distal visible part of the internal carotid artery (ICA), in transverse and gray scale (B mode). Refer to Note 1 above for rationale.

2. Start your documentation:
   a. At the common carotid artery (CCA), document anatomy, pathology (or lack of), and velocities at the proximal, mid, and distal CCA.
   b. At the level of the mid CCA, when in longitudinal view, angle the transducer more posterior and examine the vertebral artery by Doppler (and color or power Doppler if necessary).
   c. Examine the bulb or bifurcation area (a typical bulb, defined as a dilatation of the area proximal or within either vessel of the bifurcation, may not always be present) in transverse and longitudinal views. Note pathology or lack of pathology.
   d. Determine the position of the ICA and external carotid artery (ECA).
   e. Examine the ECA by Doppler (and color or power Doppler if necessary) at or near the origin of the vessel.
   f. Examine the ICA by Doppler (and color or power Doppler if necessary) at its origin and the mid and distal cervical portion.

3. Additional documentation:

 a. On plaque (location, amount, and appearance)

 b. On stenosis, by Doppler (and color or power Doppler if necessary) proximal, mid, and distal to the stenosis

 c. On anatomic variants

 d. On intervention, like stents or endarterectomy

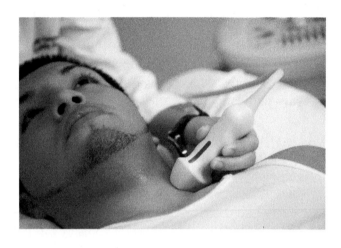

FIGURE 2.9. An example of a position of the transducer in transverse at the base of the neck. Note that, with the transducer placed on the left side of the neck, the notch of the transducer is directed toward the right side of the body. This orientation should be kept whether you are examining the right or the left side.

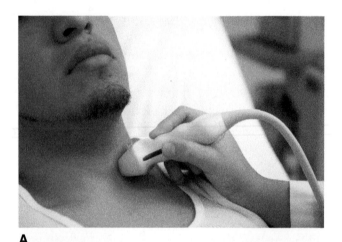

A

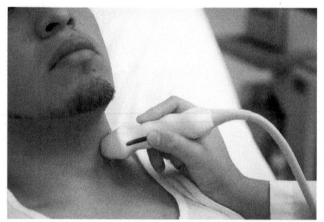

B

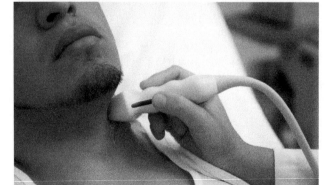

C

FIGURE 2.10. An example of a transverse sweep on the left side of the neck. The exam starts at the base of the neck and the transducer is moved cephalad (toward the head) until you reach the ICA/ECA bifurcation.

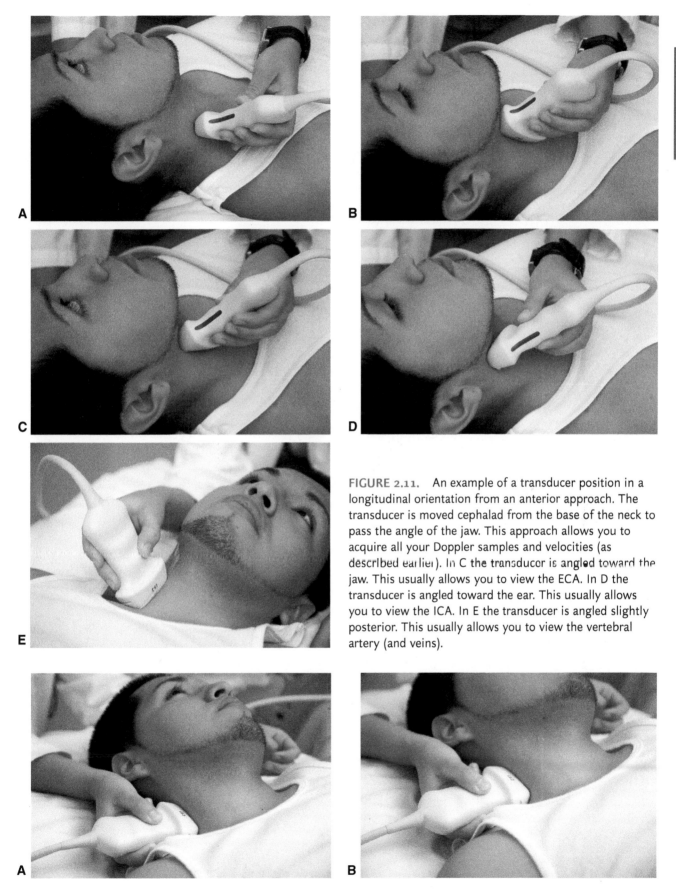

FIGURE 2.11. An example of a transducer position in a longitudinal orientation from an anterior approach. The transducer is moved cephalad from the base of the neck to pass the angle of the jaw. This approach allows you to acquire all your Doppler samples and velocities (as described earlier). In C the transducer is angled toward the jaw. This usually allows you to view the ECA. In D the transducer is angled toward the ear. This usually allows you to view the ICA. In E the transducer is angled slightly posterior. This usually allows you to view the vertebral artery (and veins).

FIGURE 2.12. Example of transducer's position from a more posterior approach. This technique may be necessary in patients with a larger neck or in patients with a surgical dressing on the neck.

Results and Interpretation on Normal Exam

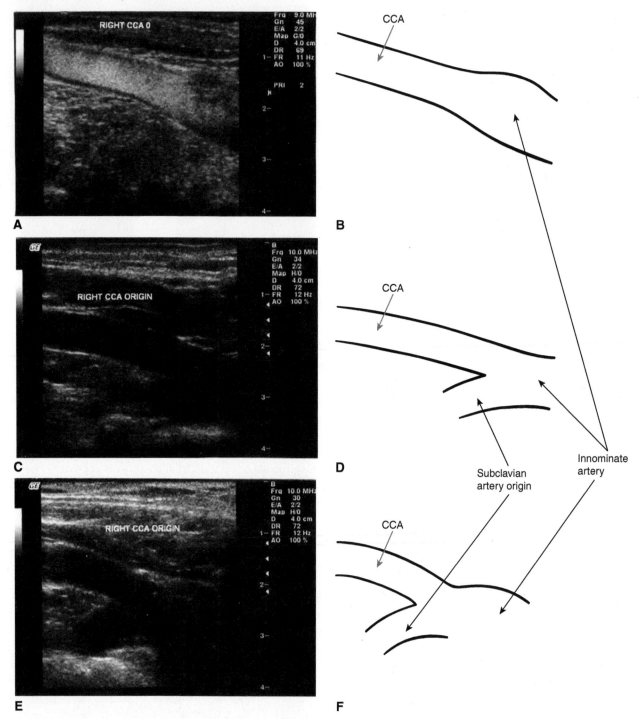

FIGURE 2.13.   Examples of CCA origin from an anterior approach (transducer notch pointing cephalad) with a longitudinal view. In A the flow is shown with B-flow (a feature available in GE equipment).

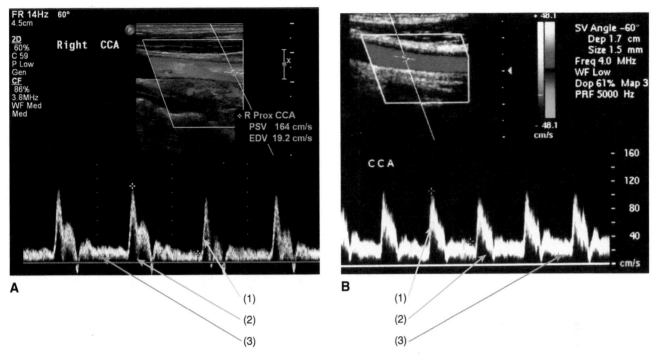

FIGURE 2.14. Normal CCA pulsed Doppler waveforms. Doppler cursor is positioned at mid stream, with a small sample gate and a Doppler angle of 60°. Transducer is positioned at the base of the neck with transducer notch pointing cephalad, anterior approach, longitudinal view. (1) Sharp upstroke in systole; (2) clear Doppler window; and (3) diastolic flow (resistance between typical ICA and ECA).

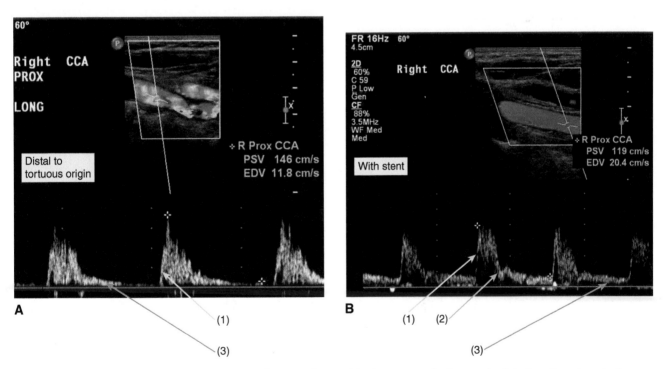

FIGURE 2.15. Other normal CCA pulsed Doppler waveforms. (1) Sharp upstroke in systole; (2) clear Doppler window; and (3) diastolic flow (resistance between typical ICA and ECA) and no plaque or narrowing.

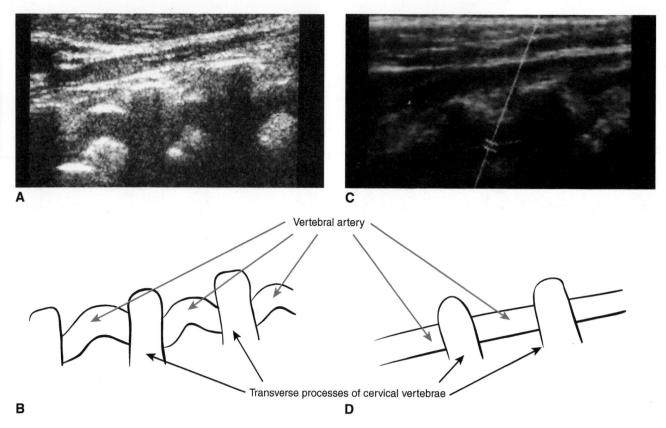

FIGURE 2.16. Examples of vertebral arteries from an anterior approach (transducer notch pointing cephalad) and in longitudinal view. The transducer will be angled slightly posterior from the position used to view the CCA.

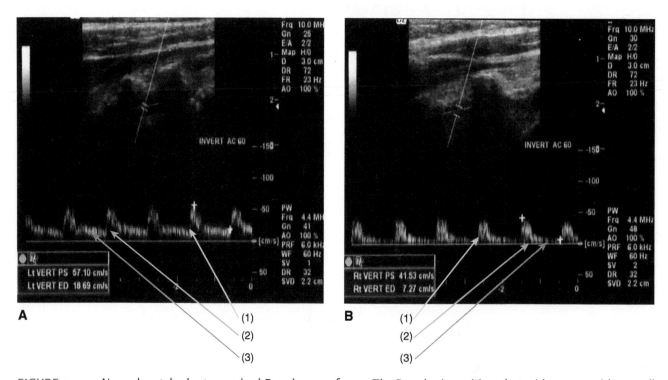

FIGURE 2.17. Normal vertebral artery pulsed Doppler waveforms. The Doppler is positioned at mid stream, with a small sample gate and a Doppler angle of 60°. (1) Sharp upstroke in systole; (2) clear Doppler window; and (3) diastolic flow (resistance between ICA and ECA); flow direction is antegrade.

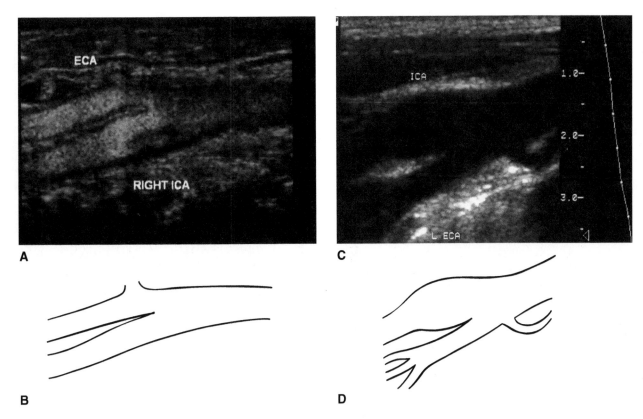

FIGURE 2.18. Distinction of the ICA from the ECA by anatomic position. In figures A and B, the ECA is usually superior (or more superficial) to the ICA from an anterior approach. In figures C and D, the ICA is now superior (or more superficial) then the ECA from a posterior approach. Caution: Independent of the approach, the relative position of the ICA and ECA can sometimes be reversed from what is typically described here. The distinction of the ICA from the ECA can therefore not rely solely on the anatomical positions of these arteries. Pulsed Doppler spectrum and presence or absence of branches will also be used to distinguish these two vessels from one another.

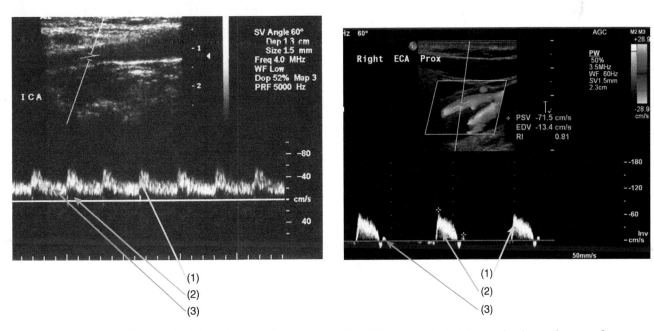

FIGURE 2.19. Typical ICA pulsed Doppler waveforms. The Doppler sample is small, placed at mid stream, and has an angle of 60°. (1) Sharp upstroke in systole; (2) clear Doppler window; and (3) high diastolic flow demonstrating low resistance.

FIGURE 2.20. Typical ECA pulsed Doppler waveforms. The Doppler sample is small, placed at mid stream, and has an angle of 60°. (1) Sharp upstroke in systole; (2) clear Doppler window; and (3) low to no diastolic flow, demonstrating high resistance.

Results and Interpretation, Normal Variants

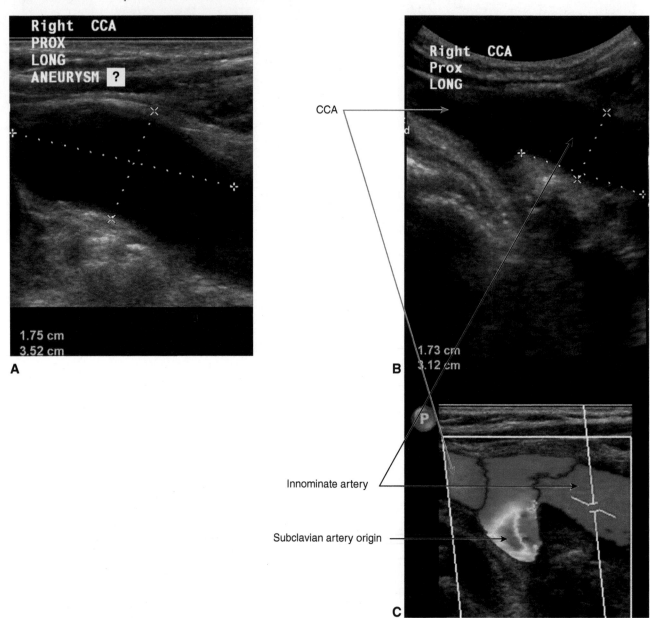

FIGURE 2.21. Unusual origin of the CCA mimicking at first glance an aneurismal dilatation. This represents an anatomical variant of a high take-off of the CCA from the brachiocephalic trunk.

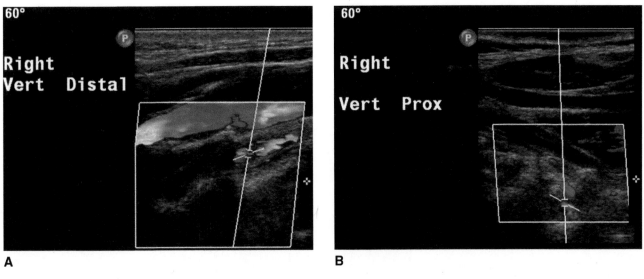

FIGURE 2.22. The vessel seen in this picture was labeled as vertebral artery. As mentioned earlier, the vertebral artery is usually best seen by angling the transducer more posteriorly when on a longitudinal view of the CCA. With such movement, the CCA is usually removed from view. In this picture, the CCA is still visible. The artery depicted may very well be a branch of the ECA or thyrocervical trunk.

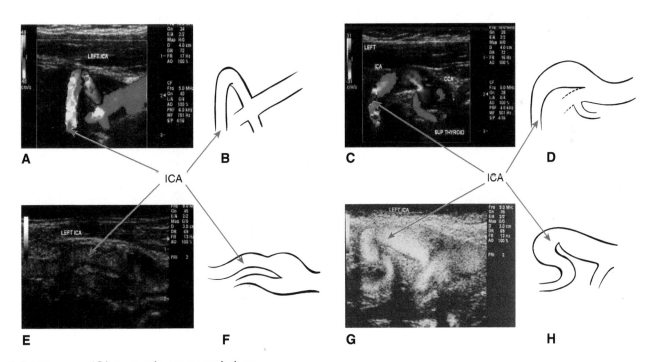

FIGURE 2.23. ICA anatomic course variations.

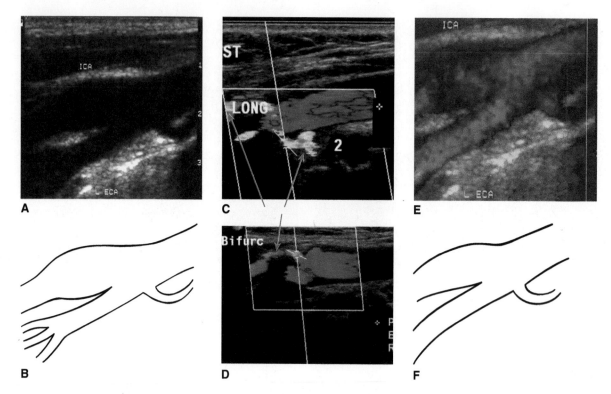

FIGURE 2.24.   Use caution in distinguishing the ICA and ECA from anatomical attributes such as branches. In figures A and B, several branches are identifiable in one vessel (the scan was probably obtained from a posterior approach) which is almost certainly the ECA. In figures C and D, the course of the branch is difficult to follow. In this case, the sonographer determined (confirmed by angiogram) that the branch was taking off the ICA. In figures E and F, the only branch seen is rather low and proximal to the ICA/ECA bifurcation. At this point positive identification of either the ICA or ECA should be done with caution and supplemental information.

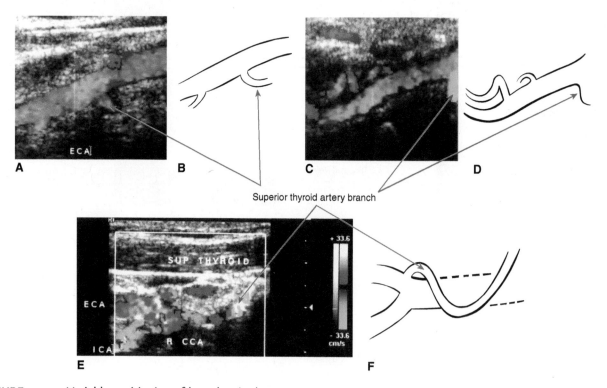

FIGURE 2.25.   Variable positioning of branches in the ECA.

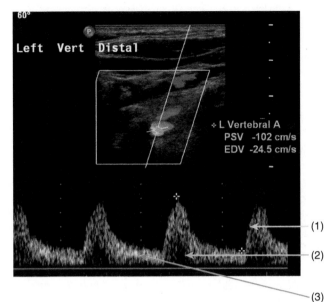

FIGURE 2.26. Normal vertebral artery Doppler with higher velocities. The flow velocities here appear slightly higher than expected, although the waveforms are normal. In this case, the ipsilateral CCA is occluded. The vertebral artery may be compensating for flow. (1) Sharp upstroke in systole; (2) clear Doppler window; and (3) diastolic flow (resistance between ICA and ECA); flow direction is antegrade.

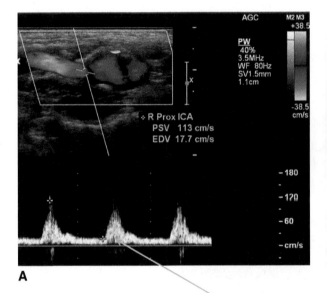

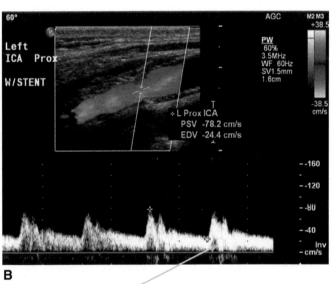

FIGURE 2.27. Normal ICA Doppler spectrum with a twist: Sharp upstroke in systole; Doppler window (arrow) filled because of turbulence from tortuous origin or large bulb (A), or because of changes in hemodynamics as with a stent (B); diastolic flow with low resistance; and no plaque.

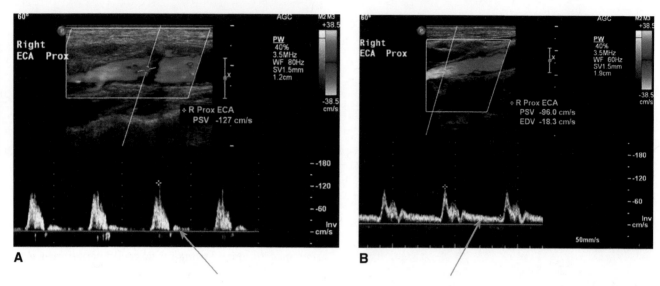

FIGURE 2.28.   Normal ECA Doppler spectrum with a twist: Sharp upstroke in systole; clear Doppler window; and diastolic flow (arrow). Although the diastolic flow appears higher than in figure 2.20, these waveforms still demonstrate high resistance compared to ICA or even CCA waveforms.

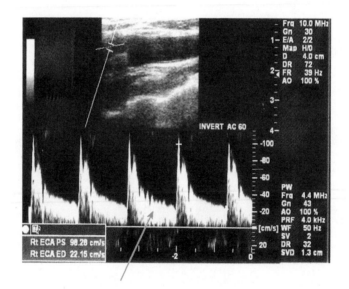

FIGURE 2.29.   Normal ECA Doppler waveform with temporal tap (arrow). This maneuver is performed by gently and rapidly tapping the temple with one finger while insonating the ECA with Doppler. The "taps" are recorded with small and rhythmic changes in the waveforms as shown here. Temporal tap is one maneuver allowing distinction between ICA and ECA. The ICA usually does not display changes in spectral Doppler with a temporal tap but it could. Use the temporal tap with caution.

Results and Interpretation, Abnormal and Pathology Findings

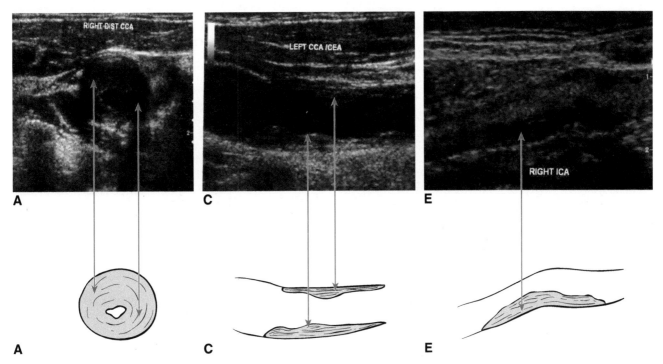

FIGURE 2.30. The plaques here are echolucent and mostly homogeneous. These plaques are usually "soft" plaques without much fibrous material. They are usually unstable and can be the source of emboli. Flow in E is depicted with B flow.

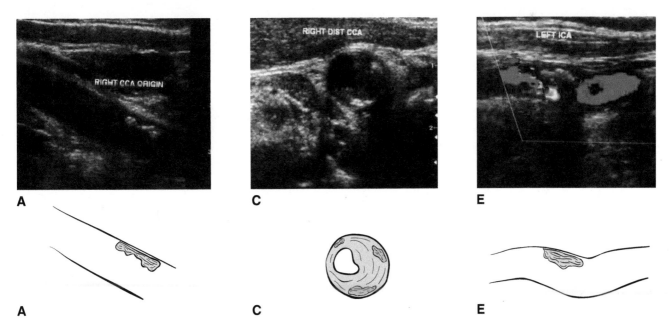

FIGURE 2.31. The plaques here are echogenic and mostly heterogeneous. These plaques are usually "hard" and contain some calcification as well as fibrous material. These plaques tend to be more stable.

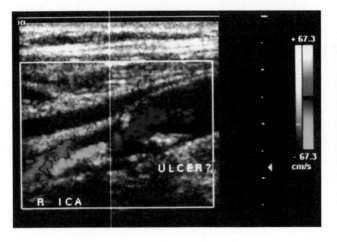

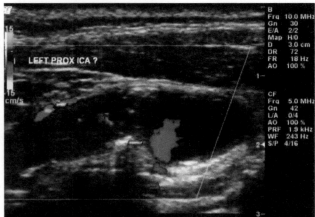

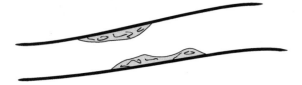

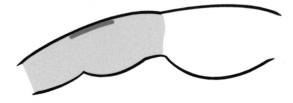

FIGURE 2.32. Probable ulcer with crater. The patient here had symptoms of right eye amaurosis fugax for 6 months prior to exam. The patient underwent a carotid endarterectomy the next day. The pathologic examination of the specimen revealed ulceration.

FIGURE 2.33. Possible "string sign" in this proximal ICA. The stenosis is, at this point, so critical that the velocities have dropped dramatically.

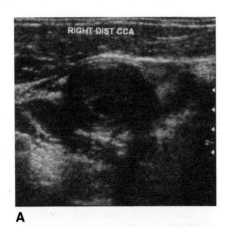

A

B

% Stenosis by area:

$(1 - x/y)^2 \times 100 = \%$ Area reduction

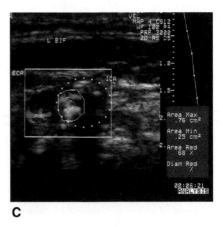

C

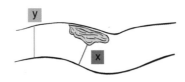

D   **E**

% Stenosis by diameter:

$(y - x/y) \times 100 = \%$ Diameter reduction

FIGURE 2.34. Determining stenosis by directly measuring the narrowing.

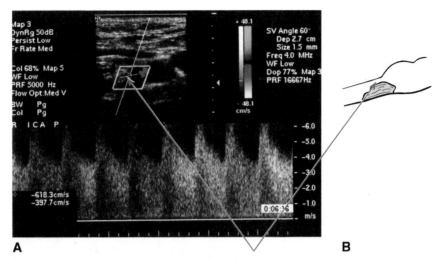

FIGURE 2.35. Determining stenosis "indirectly" by recording flow velocities. The Doppler sample is in the mid stream of the narrowest portion (as much as possible) of the stenosis and with an angle of 60° or less. In this example, the velocities are recorded at > 600 cm/s in peak systole and almost 400 cm/s in end diastole. These would correspond to a critical stenosis of the proximal ICA with all diagnosis criteria used for this type of exam.

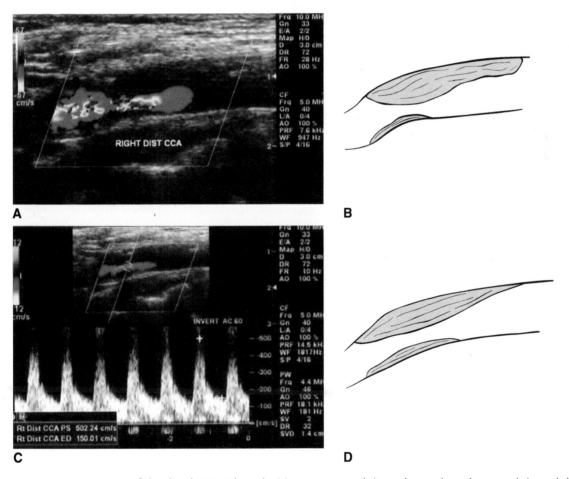

FIGURE 2.36. Severe stenosis of the distal CCA. The velocities are 500 cm/s in peak systole and 150 cm/s in end diastole. Even though we do not have the velocities at a more proximal nondiseased segment, normal CCA velocities are not generally higher than 130 cm/s in peak systole. In this case, 500 cm/s represents more than a doubling of velocities and, therefore, a greater than 50% stenosis.

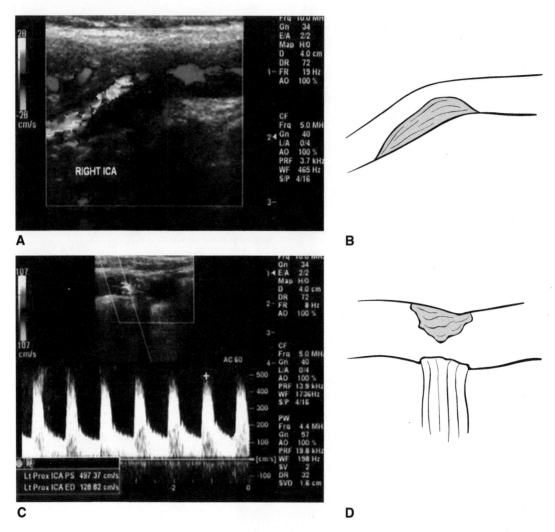

FIGURE 2.37.   Severe stenosis of the proximal ICA. The velocities are > 450 cm/s in peak systole and 130 cm/s in end diastole.

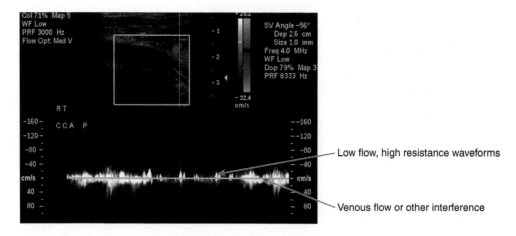

FIGURE 2.38.   In this picture, the flow is visible by color Doppler, and the pulsed Doppler waveforms display low flow with very high resistance, which can be seen proximal to an occlusion. Power Doppler could have been used here to display some of the low flow. In this case the velocity scale should also have been lowered for better analysis of the Doppler spectrum. This is a good example of poor optimization or use of tools on the equipment.

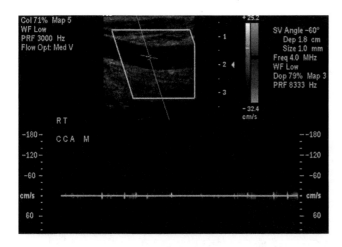

FIGURE 2.39.   Occluded vessel is shown, and no color fill or pulsed Doppler spectrum is displayed. Note: As a precaution and to avoid missing a "string sign" or very low flow, the spectral range could have been decreased further to 10 cm/s, or power Doppler could have been used. Another example of poor optimization or use of tools on the equipment.

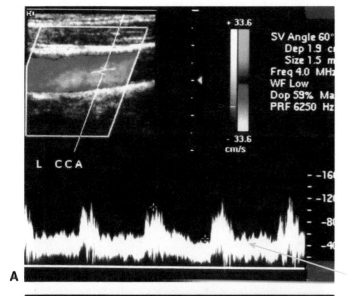

A

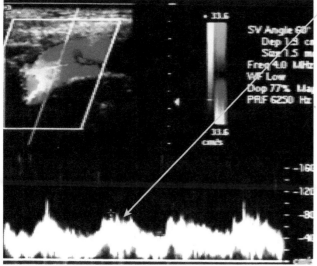

B

FIGURE 2.40.   Example of turbulence on a CCA and an ICA Doppler spectrum without evidence of plaque. This patient had a known intracranial arteriovenous malformation. This type of observation shows the versatility of the evaluation of the extracranial circulation where much more distal problems can already be evident in the hemodynamics of the vessels of the neck.

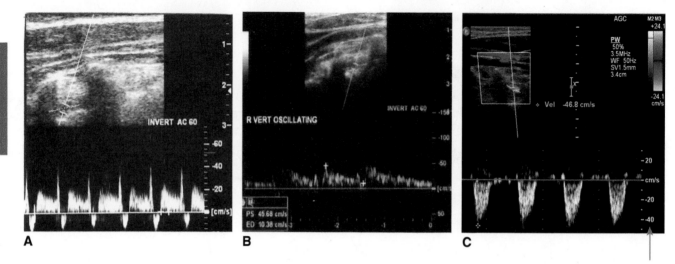

FIGURE 2.41. Samples of vertebral arteries pulsed Doppler waveforms in the presence of subclavian steal phenomenon. (A) The flow spectrum is very briefly antegrade in the beginning of systole; then, it is displayed as positive with this spectral Doppler setting, demonstrating here a short reversal of flow; this is followed by normal antegrade flow, shown as negative on the flow spectrum. Seen with partial steal. (B) Oscillating flow as described in the previous image with less pronounced retrograde flow in late systole. Seen with partial steal. (C) Complete reversal of flow. The flow is retrograde throughout the cardiac cycle in this image, where the Doppler spectrum is shown as negative (arrow) when it should be positive in regard to the position of the Doppler sample.

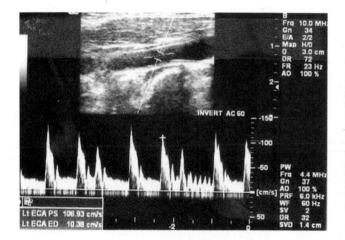

FIGURE 2.42. Irregular heart rhythm apparent in an ECA pulsed Doppler waveforms. Note the rhythm: one peak followed by two shorter peaks at reduced distance.

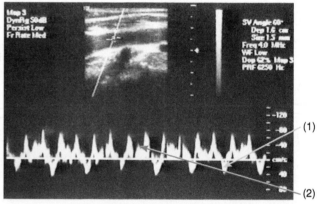

FIGURE 2.43. Irregular rhythm apparent in a CCA pulsed Doppler waveform. The patient was on an intra-aortic balloon pump. The balloon is inflated during early diastole and delivers counterpulsation or augmentation. It then deflates just prior to systolic ejection, resulting in decreased intra-aortic pressure. (1) Deflation prior to systolic ejection results in slight reversal of flow. (2) Inflation during early diastole results in Doppler spectrum peak in late diastole.

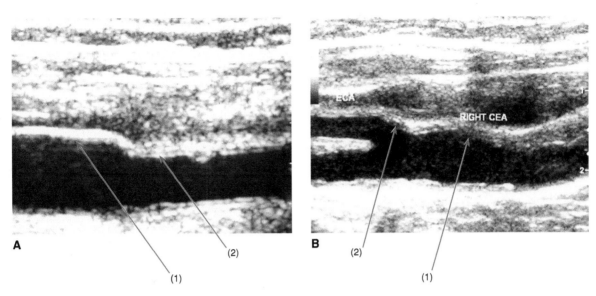

FIGURE 2.44.   Samples of ICAs after a carotid endarterectomy. Note the absence of intima at the level of the endarterectomy sites (1), as well as the slightly enlarged lumen probably due to the apposition of a patch for closure of the endarterectomy sites. (2) Intima in native vessel.

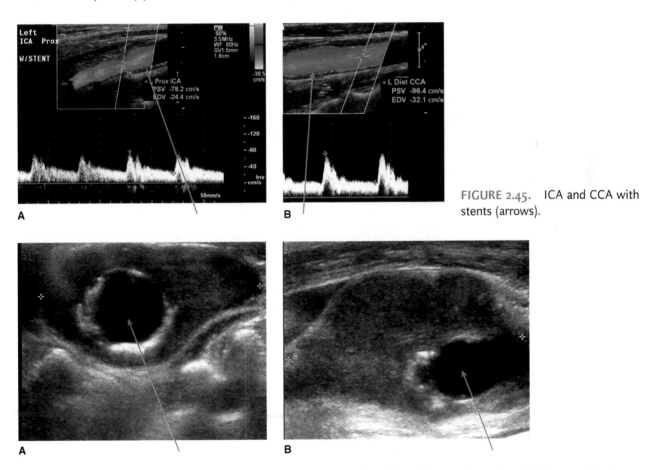

FIGURE 2.45.   ICA and CCA with stents (arrows).

FIGURE 2.46.   An example of a carotid body tumor transverse view (A) and longitudinal view (B). The carotid glomus or glomus caroticum is located in the region of the distal common carotid and/or carotid bifurcation, as a small ovoid mass containing chemoreceptors for the regulation of oxygen in the arterial blood. Transformation to a tumor is usually benign although it can induce symptoms of dysphagia when the tumor is enlarged. A biopsy is not recommended due to high vascularization. Surgical excision is the typical treatment. Courtesy of Philips.

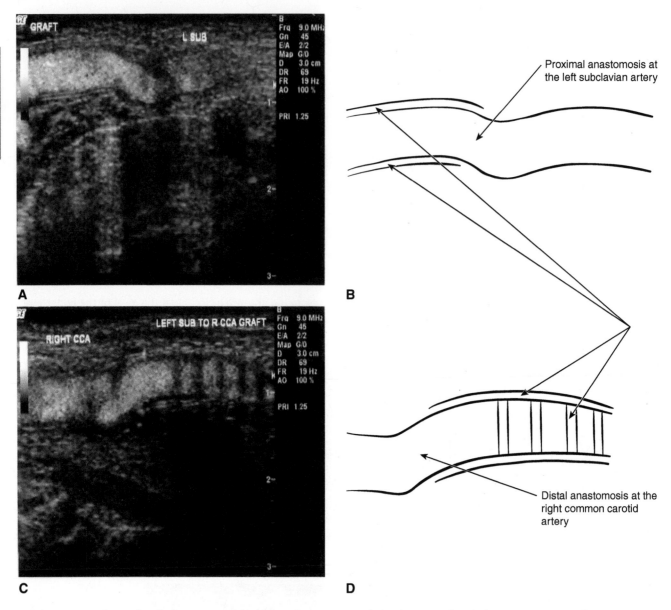

FIGURE 2.47. Example of a bypass graft involving the extracranial circulation. Left subclavian artery to right CCA bypass graft with Gortex. The graft was probably positioned to bypass an innominate artery occlusion. The flow is depicted with B flow in these pictures. The shadows and thick lines are characteristics of synthetic grafts.

Concluding Tips

- Do not become a slave to numbers.
- Correlate what you see (plaque or other) with what you get (velocities) and with what you know (patient history, age, physical condition, and symptoms).
- The carotid artery system, particularly the ICA, follows a rather complicated embryologic development where arteries appear, recede, and merge to form the final ICA. Anatomic variants are relatively rare but very real! If a vessel seems out of place or missing, then it probably is; an abnormality is not necessarily a result of occlusion.

- Because of this embryologic development, many collateral routes are possible, so understand, document, and report any observed changes in direction of flow from what is expected.
- When in doubt, ask for help, suggest another test, inquire about the results, and document and perhaps publish your findings.

General Concepts for the Extracranial Venous Circulation

The extracranial circulation also includes major venous channels, and this chapter would not be complete without discussing their evaluation by ultrasound. Indeed, for those practicing or looking forward to practicing in hospital settings, a clear understanding of the proper evaluation of the jugular venous system will be an asset. Advances in medicine and treatments have required an increasing use of indwelling catheters through major accessible veins, such as the internal jugular vein. These catheters or lines inserted in all veins have also introduced a new array of complications such as thrombosis (mainly) of veins that are not naturally prone to thrombosis, such as the internal jugular vein.

Tips/Rationale

The examination of the internal jugular vein can be done:

- As an incidental examination during an extracranial carotid artery system evaluation
- As a specific request, because of increased swelling to the face and neck, generally after catheterization of intravenous cannulation (for multiple reasons)
- As part of the evaluation of the venous system of the upper extremity (see Chapter 4)
- For very particular reasons/requests such as:
  - Trauma to the neck, with suspicion of arteriovenous fistula
  - Difficult cannulation of the vessel

Protocol Algorithm

There is really no accepted protocol (or sole billing code) for evaluation of the extracranial (or intracranial for that matter) venous circulation by itself and for other reasons than those mentioned earlier. The only protocol where the internal jugular vein is mentioned is the one pertinent to the assessment of the upper extremity venous system.

Duplex Exam of the Extracranial Venous Circulation

Test Preparation

Follow similar imaging techniques as those described for the evaluation of the extracranial carotid artery system. The main exception will be in case of indication for examination following insertion of a catheter or other device

CHAPTER 2

temporarily placed in the vessel's lumen. In this case, the device will probably be held in place by bandages and/or surgical tape. Removal of the tape and bandage is not recommended. Most patients requiring catheterization or an intravenous (IV) line through the jugular vein are receiving either chemotherapy or hemodialysis and are very immunologically fragile. The exam can still be performed by adopting any approach that could circumvent the bandage or, in cases where the physician or nurse has authorized the removal of the dressing, by applying a sterile coupling film before scanning the area.

Test Sequence

There is no particular or prescribed test sequence. However, as with the carotid system, the exam should probably and most logically start at the base of the neck with the transducer held in a transverse fashion. This would be followed by a longitudinal approach for examination with pulsed Doppler.

Results and Interpretation

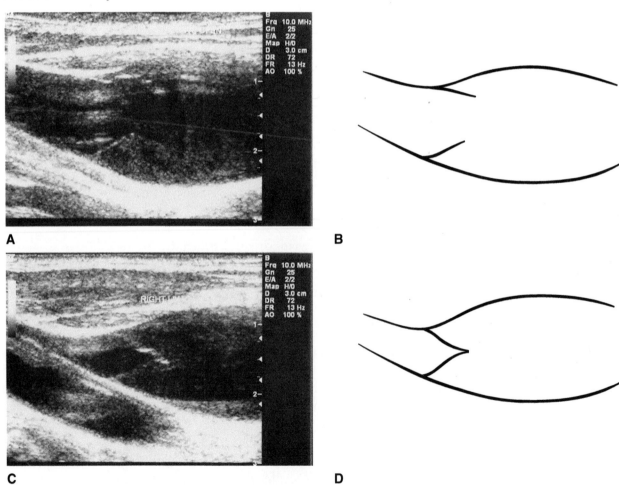

FIGURE 2.48.   Valves (A and B, open; C and D, closed) in the internal jugular vein at the junction with the brachiocephalic trunk. Note: The slightly echoic material seen in the valve cusps does not represent thrombosis but the "rouleaux" effect visible even with two-dimensional imaging due to slow flow and turbulence in veins.

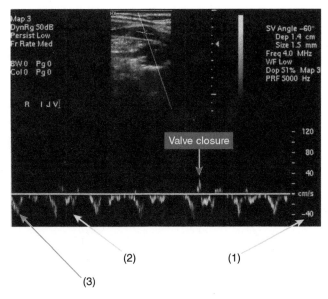

FIGURE 2.49. Normal Doppler spectrum in the internal jugular vein. The Doppler sample is small, placed at mid stream, and has an angle of 60°. Note: Although using a correct Doppler angle to insonate veins is not crucial (because we do not use velocity criteria for diagnosis), adding a correct position of cursor and Doppler angle allows for future comparison of exams if pathology was to develop. Typical internal jugular vein waveforms (with pulsed wave Doppler): (1) flow is retrograde (toward the heart); (2) flow is phasic with respiration (represented by slight oscillation in the Doppler wave); and (3) flow is pulsatile due to the proximity of the heart. Changes in the Doppler spectrum of the internal jugular can point to partial or total occlusion of the innominate veins or superior vena cava, which are difficult to visualize by ultrasound. These could show loss of phasicity and pulsatility.

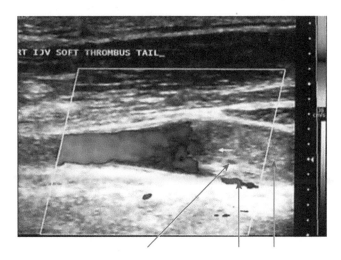

FIGURE 2.50. Thrombosis of the internal jugular vein. Thrombus is getting organized (seen by the level of echoes) and retracted (seen by some flow between the intima and thrombus).

Concluding Tips

Although the internal jugular vein is not naturally prone to disease, the examination of that vessel during a carotid exam or for specific unexplained symptoms may reveal information. Be vigilant and thorough when documenting results in this vessel.

PART TWO: UPPER EXTREMITIES

Testing the Arterial Circulation

Chapter Outline

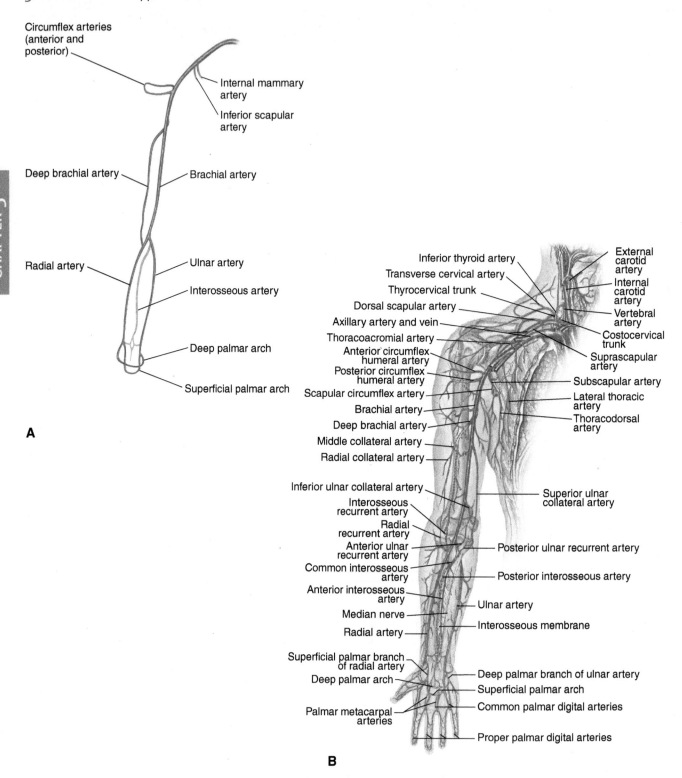

FIGURE 3.1. Anterior view of the arterial system of the upper extremity in anatomic position.

General Concepts in Upper Extremity Arterial Evaluation

The upper extremity arterial system should be considered from its inflow, at the level of the subclavian artery on the left and the brachiocephalic trunk or innominate artery on the right, to its distal portion at the levels of the digits.

It is worth noting that in regard to the pathologic processes involving the arteries of the upper extremities, the system could be divided into three separate and somewhat distinct portions:

- The first portion includes the levels of the clavicle, shoulder, and axilla, with the inflow arteries: innominate, subclavian and axillary arteries.
- The second portion includes the arm and forearm, with the brachial, deep brachial, radial, and ulnar arteries.
- The third portion consists of the hand, with the palmar arches and digital arteries.

Each portion seems to be predominantly affected by discrete pathologic phenomena, such as:

- First Portion:
  - Typical atherosclerotic disease (with the left side being affected more often than the right, thought to be a result of the anatomic take off of the left subclavian at a sharp angle from the aortic arch).
  - Inflammatory processes of the larger arteries such as Takayasu's disease (which should be suspected in young females in the second or third decade with upper extremity claudication or ischemia or decreased pulses or blood pressure).
  - Mechanical compression, such as thoracic outlet syndrome.

- Second Portion:
  - Medial calcification (another form of arteriosclerosis) of the radial and/or ulnar artery is sometimes seen in patients with type 1 diabetes mellitus (with similar presentation as in the tibial vessels) and in patients on hemodialysis with an upper extremity access.
  - Anatomic variants at the level of the bifurcation of the brachial artery into the radial and ulnar arteries, although not pathologic processes per se, can trigger potential problems. These are particularly important when evaluating patency of the palmar arches before insertion of a hemodialysis access.

- Third Portion:
  - Buerger's disease, which is still mostly of unknown etiology, will affect the digits of the hands and also feet.
  - Increased sensitivity to cold or other vasospastic phenomena, such as Raynaud's disease.

Tips/Rationale

As with many of our examinations in the vascular laboratory, the rationale for evaluating upper extremity arterial circulation will be linked to understanding, if not the etiology, at least the source or potential source of the symptoms. As such, and ideally, we would need to proceed through the following different steps:

- Determine whether the origin of the pain is of vascular origin versus neurologic or musculoskeletal by the medical history and presentation of symptoms.
- Perform a physiologic test at rest as the primary test to obtain an overall understanding.
- Add maneuvers or exercise if the pain seems to be triggered by positioning of the upper extremity, as would be seen with mechanical compression (at the thoracic outlet).
- And/or perform a duplex ultrasound evaluation of the inflow arteries and the carotid/vertebral system if inflow disease is suspected.
- And/or evaluate the perfusion of the digits if the symptoms are localized at that level and no other restrictions of flow are noted more proximally.

Protocol Algorithm

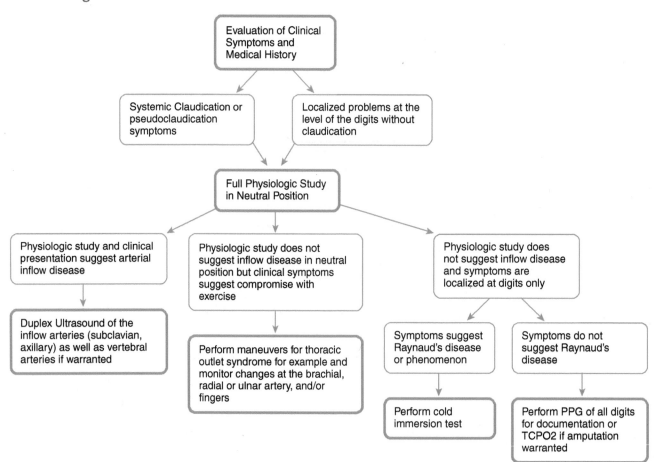

FIGURE 3.2. Examination algorithm for the upper extremity arterial circulation.

Examination of the Upper Extremity Arterial Circulation

Test Preparation

The test preparation for any of the exams of the upper extremities entails only a few points, as described below:

■ The physiologic test at rest and, as much as possible, the duplex exam should be performed with the patient supine and the upper extremities resting comfortably in a neutral position at the same level as the heart.

■ The room should be warm and the atmosphere relaxing.

■ The test should start with a thorough medical history, including very important lifestyle factors such as smoking, leisure, or professional activities.

■ Any extra testing that entails maneuvers will be better performed with the patient sitting. It is easier in a sitting position to perform the maneuvers for thoracic outlet syndrome, and it ensure a better positioning of the photoplethysmography (PPG) leads for Raynaud's syndrome or other evaluation of the circulation of the digits.

Testing Sequence

Physiologic Studies at Rest

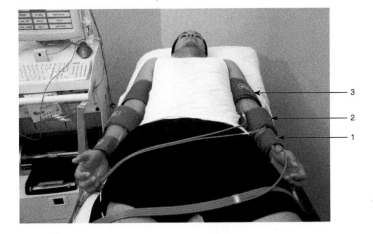

FIGURE 3.3.   Pulse volume recording (PVR) sequence. The number represents the chronological sequence of inflation of the cuffs. Starting at the wrist and moving proximally is ideal. Remember to perform bilateral exam.

CHAPTER 3

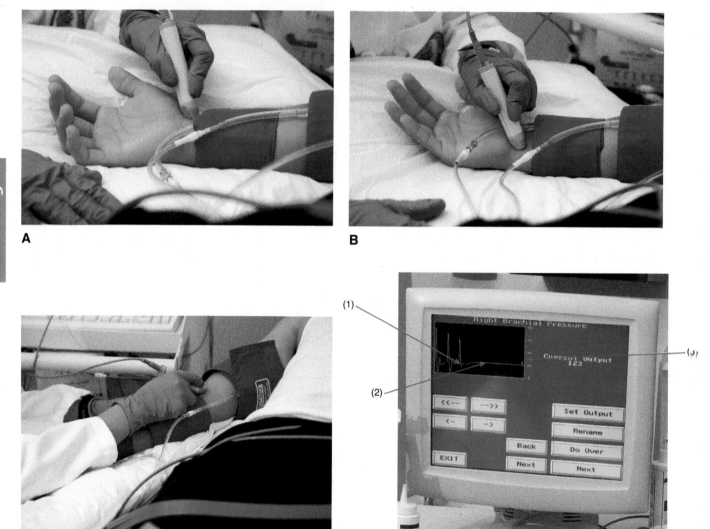

FIGURE 3.4.   Segmental pressures sequence.

As with PVR, it is recommended to take the first pressures at the wrist to avoid reactive hyperemia with cuff inflation first at the branchial level. Photo D shows the monitor display to illustrate the process of obtaining pressure by Doppler. With the CW Doppler continuously on the artery, the inflation of the cuff is stopped once the signal disappears (1). The cuff is then deflated slowly, at a rate of approximately 2 mmHg per heart beat (2). The reappearance of the signal marks the systolic pressure at that level (in the vessel under the cuff) (3).

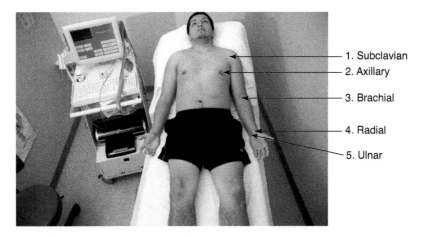

FIGURE 3.5. Continuous wave (CW) Doppler data. There is no specific need for a particular sequence to be followed in obtaining CW waveforms. For ease the cuffs have been removed so this part is often done first or last. However the CW Doppler waveforms can also be obtained with the cuffs in place as seen in Figure 3.4 and before obtaining pressures. The CW Doppler will be placed with an angle of 60 degrees or less between the transducer and the course of the vessel as illustrated in Figures 3.4A through C.

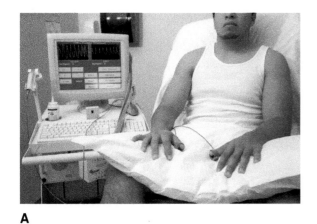

A

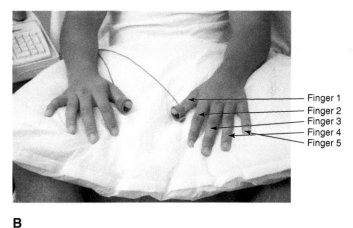

B

FIGURE 3.6. PPG waveforms sequence at room temperature for baseline data. The leads will be moved bilaterally from the first to fifth fingers.

CHAPTER 3

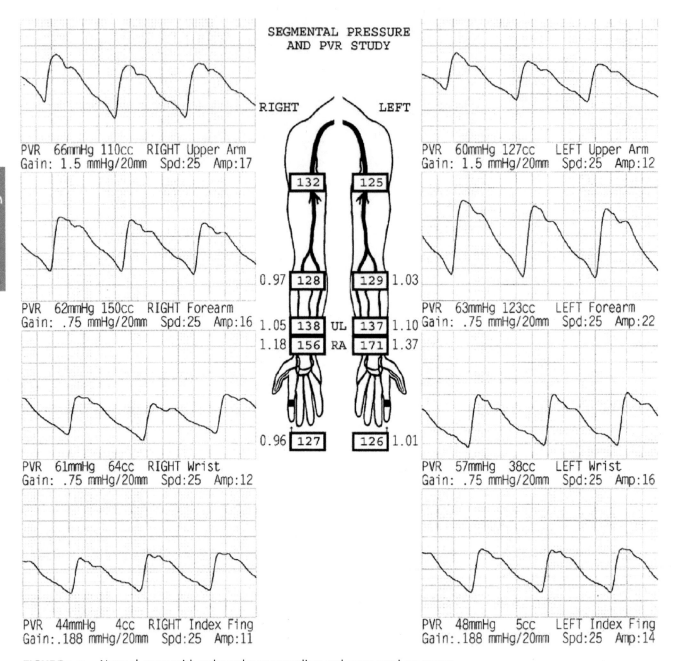

SEGMENTAL PRESSURE
AND PVR STUDY

RIGHT   LEFT

PVR 66mmHg 110cc RIGHT Upper Arm
Gain: 1.5 mmHg/20mm Spd:25 Amp:17

PVR 60mmHg 127cc   LEFT Upper Arm
Gain: 1.5 mmHg/20mm Spd:25 Amp:12

132   125

PVR 62mmHg 150cc RIGHT Forearm
Gain: .75 mmHg/20mm Spd:25 Amp:16

PVR 63mmHg 123cc   LEFT Forearm
Gain: .75 mmHg/20mm Spd:25 Amp:22

0.97 128   129 1.03

1.05 138 UL 137 1.10
1.18 156 RA 171 1.37

PVR 61mmHg 64cc RIGHT Wrist
Gain: .75 mmHg/20mm Spd:25 Amp:12

PVR 57mmHg 38cc LEFT Wrist
Gain: .75 mmHg/20mm Spd:25 Amp:16

0.96 127   126 1.01

PVR 44mmHg 4cc RIGHT Index Fing
Gain:.188 mmHg/20mm Spd:25 Amp:11

PVR 48mmHg 5cc LEFT Index Fing
Gain:.188 mmHg/20mm Spd:25 Amp:14

FIGURE 3.7.   Normal exam with pulse volume recording and segmental pressures.

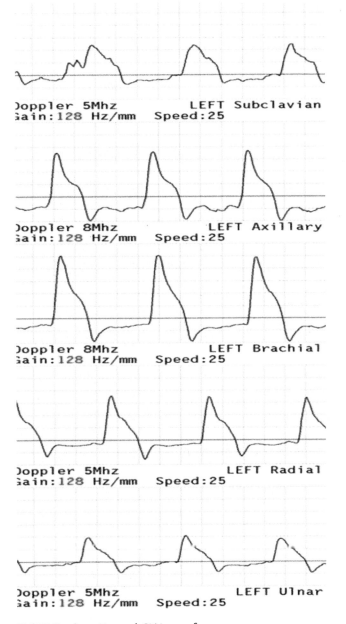

FIGURE 3.8.   Normal CW waveforms.

CHAPTER 3

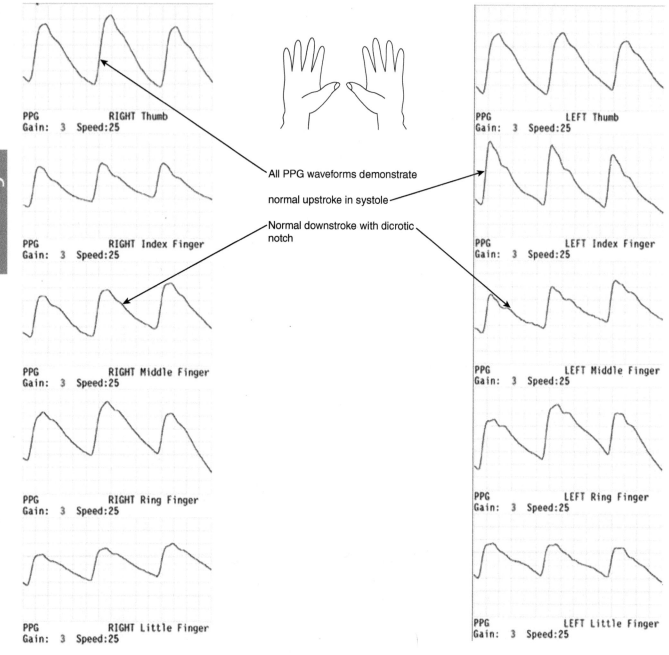

PPG   RIGHT Thumb
Gain: 3 Speed:25

All PPG waveforms demonstrate

normal upstroke in systole

Normal downstroke with dicrotic
notch

PPG   RIGHT Index Finger
Gain: 3 Speed:25

PPG   RIGHT Middle Finger
Gain: 3 Speed:25

PPG   RIGHT Ring Finger
Gain: 3 Speed:25

PPG   RIGHT Little Finger
Gain: 3 Speed:25

PPG   LEFT Thumb
Gain: 3 Speed:25

PPG   LEFT Index Finger
Gain: 3 Speed:25

PPG   LEFT Middle Finger
Gain: 3 Speed:25

PPG   LEFT Ring Finger
Gain: 3 Speed:25

PPG   LEFT Little Finger
Gain: 3 Speed:25

FIGURE 3.9.   Normal PPG waveforms at rest and room temperature.

Physiologic Studies Sequence, Special Considerations

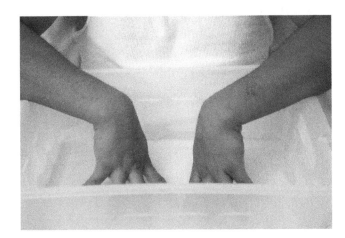

FIGURE 3.10.   To test for Raynaud's disease and/or suspected increased sensitivity to cold, data will be obtained first at room temperature, usually using PPG leads on each finger. After removing the PPG leads, the hands could then be immersed in a bucket with cold water (you may add a few ice cubes if the tap water is not too cold) for a few minutes. Pat dry the hands without re-warming and place PPG leads to obtain data. The sequence will be repeated at different time intervals until the PPG leads record baseline waveforms or until 10 minutes have passed (typical protocol).

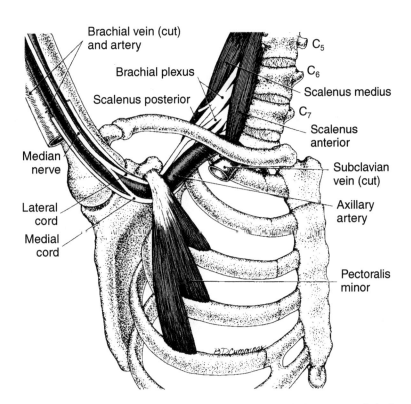

FIGURE 3.11.   The thoracic outlet is the region where the subclavian vessels (vein and artery) and the brachial nerve plexus enter the upper extremity appendage. In some cases, because of the position of the first rib, clavicle, and/or the pectoralis muscle, the vein, artery, and/or nerve can be compressed during strenuous exercises or specific maneuvers. This may lead to thrombosis in the subclavian veins or injury to the subclavian artery.

Thoracic Outlet Syndrome

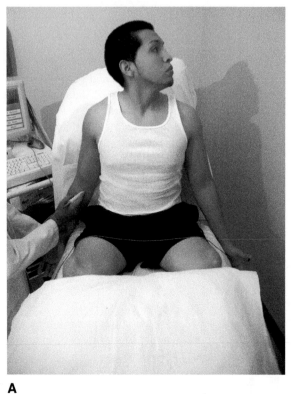

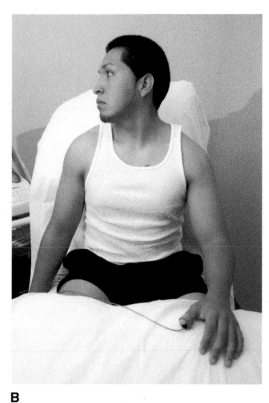

A   **B**

FIGURE 3.12. Patient performing costoclavicular compression or exaggerated military maneuver. CW Doppler at the brachial artery or PPG on first digit are maintained to evaluate changes during maneuvers.

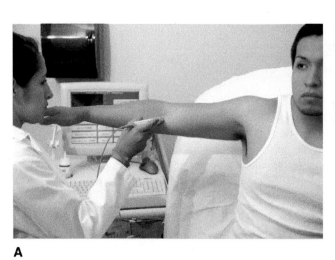

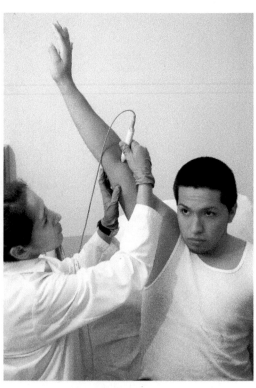

A   **B**

FIGURE 3.13. Patient performing hyperabduction. CW Doppler at the brachial artery or PPG at the first digit are maintained to evaluate changes during maneuvers. (Continued)

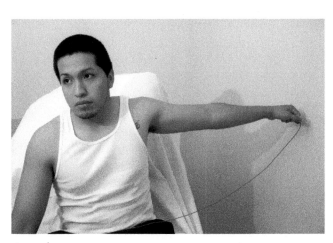

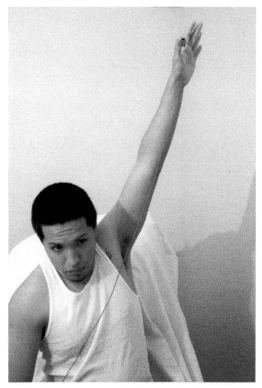

C

D

FIGURE 3.13. (Continued)

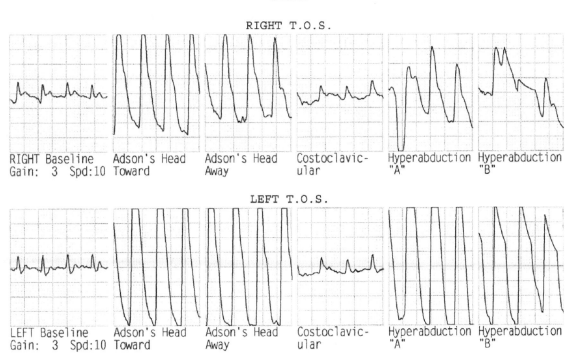

FIGURE 3.14. Results of TOS maneuvers with PPG. With CW Doppler, you want to see a continuous triphasic signal at the brachial artery. Note: The Adson's and costoclavicular maneuvers can be used independently or in combination (as in the photos). In a true Adson's maneuver, the shoulders are in neutral position and the arm raised at 90 degrees and bent at the elbow with the hand up.

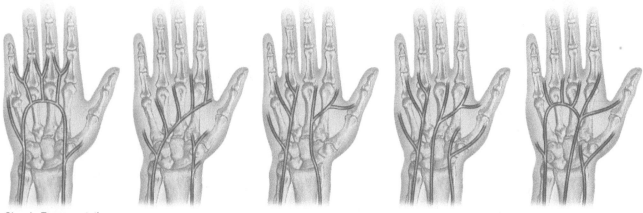

Classic Representation presents in 43% of right hand and 52% of left hand.

Most common configuration of incomplete superficial palmar arches. Those involving a median artery supplying part of the hand in addition to the ulnar and radial arteries represent approximately 10% of the variations.

FIGURE 3.15.   Variations of the superficial palmar arch. These are important points to remember when performing Allen's test.

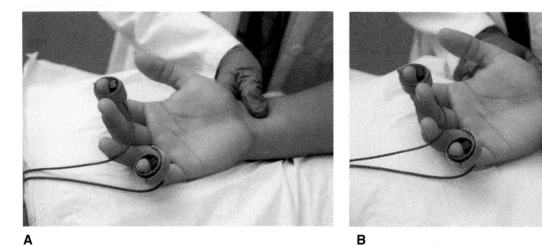

A

B

FIGURE 3.16.   Performing Allen's test with PPG leads (can also use CW Doppler at the wrist).

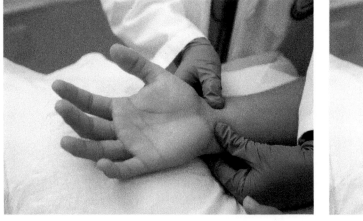

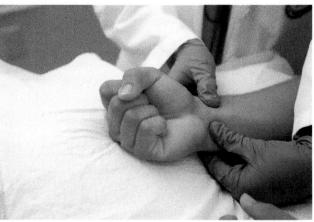

A

B

FIGURE 3.17.   Alternate technique for Allen's test. Both the ulnar and radial arteries are compressed. The patient is instructed to perform several rapid fist clenches until the hands is exsanguinated. The pressure is released alternating from the radial and ulnar. The hand is visually inspected for return of color.   (Continued)

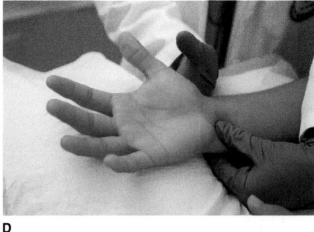
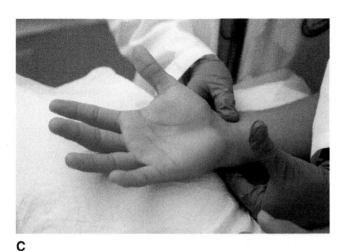

C   D

FIGURE 3.17.   (Continued)

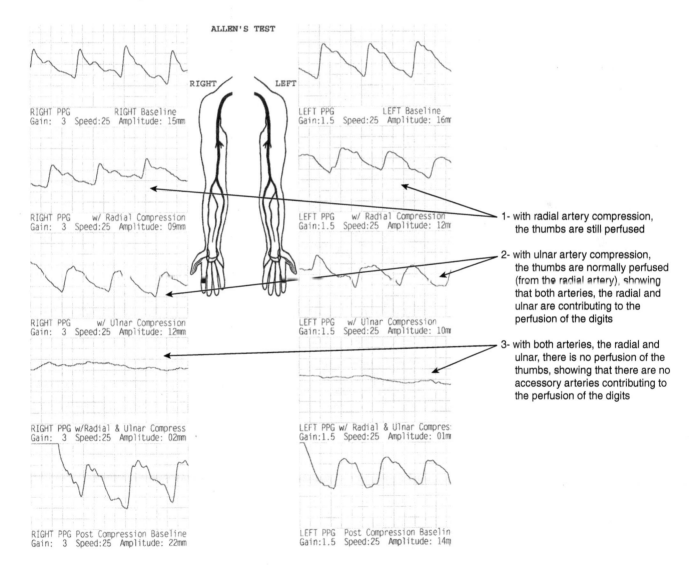

1- with radial artery compression, the thumbs are still perfused

2- with ulnar artery compression, the thumbs are normally perfused (from the radial artery), showing that both arteries, the radial and ulnar are contributing to the perfusion of the digits

3- with both arteries, the radial and ulnar, there is no perfusion of the thumbs, showing that there are no accessory arteries contributing to the perfusion of the digits

FIGURE 3.18.   Normal PPG printouts with Allen's test. Note: The sequence will vary with different physiologic equipment. The setting on the equipment should reflect and be tailored to the practice of the laboratory and the population served. Interpretation: What this test sequence is illustrating is patency of the palmar arches with the radial and ulnar arteries being the main arteries feeding the palmar arches.

Duplex Ultrasound

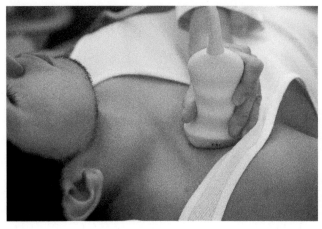

A

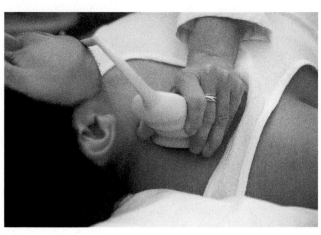

B

FIGURE 3.19.   Taking PW Doppler at the subclavian artery, two approaches. In A the transducer is placed below the clavicle with a slight superior angling. In B the transducer is placed above the clavicle pointing inferior.

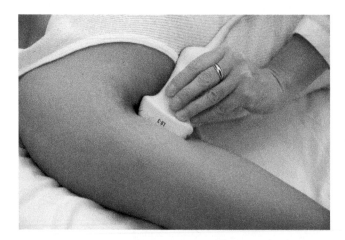

FIGURE 3.20.   Taking pulsed wave Doppler at the axillary artery.

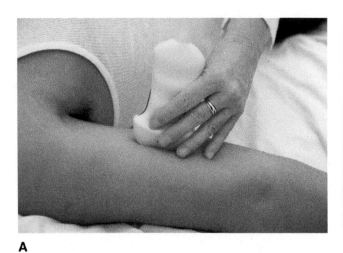

A

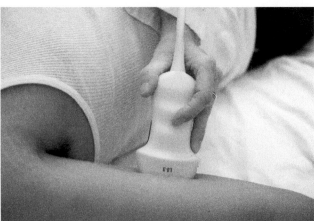

B

FIGURE 3.21.   Taking pulsed wave Doppler along the arteries of the arm and forearm.

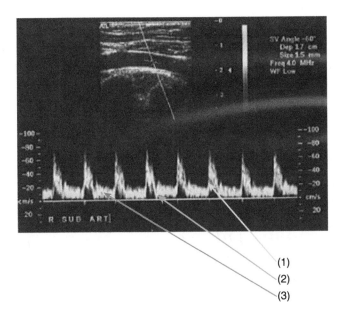

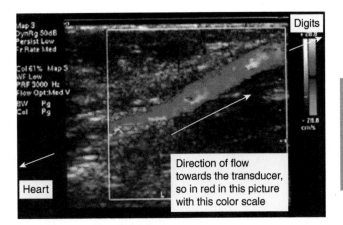

FIGURE 3.22.   Normal pulsed wave (PW) Doppler wave-forms. Typical PW Doppler spectrum in inflow arteries to the upper extremities. The waveform displays: (1) sharp upstroke in systole; (2) some reversal of flow in early diastole (high resistance); and (3) forward flow in late diastole. In this instance, there is high flow (and barely visible flow reversal) because the distal arteries are vasodilated due to the warm temperature of the room. It is not unusual to obtain high diastolic flow (showing lower resistance) in arteries of the upper extremities.

FIGURE 3.23.   Flow direction can be examined using color Doppler. This technique also allows one to evaluate the patency of the vessel.

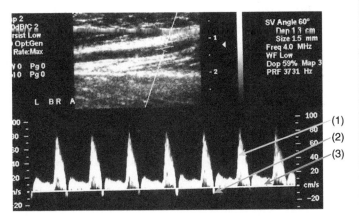

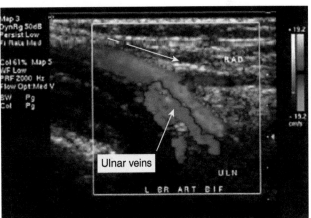

FIGURE 3.24.   Normal pulsed wave Doppler waveforms. Flow direction can also be examined using pulsed Doppler. The waveform displays: (1) sharp upstroke in systole; (2) some reversal of flow in early diastole (high resistance); and (3) forward flow in late diastole.

FIGURE 3.25.   Typical brachial artery bifurcation. Direction of flow is away from the transducer (normal) and displayed in blue in this picture with this color scale.

CHAPTER 3

Results and Interpretation

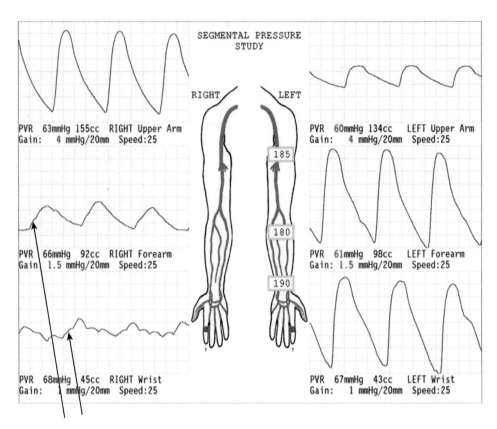

FIGURE 3.26.   Abnormal physiologic test at rest in patient with right arm claudication and signs of ischemia on a digit (and hemodialysis access graft). PPG waveforms at all digits of the right hand in this patient showed no flow (see Figure 3.27). Note the diminished flow in the forearm (arrows) evident with the rounded pulsed volume recording waveforms, showing filling delay in systole.

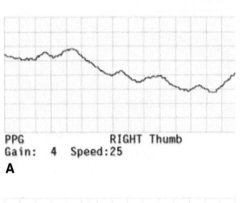

PPG   RIGHT Thumb
Gain: 4   Speed:25

A

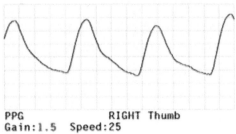

PPG   RIGHT Thumb
Gain:1.5   Speed:25

B

FIGURE 3.27.   PPG waveforms to a digit of the right hand in a patient with a hemodialysis access graft. Patient has right arm claudication and sign of ischemia on the digit. (A) PPG waveforms with hemodialysis access fully functioning. The PPG waveforms on that particular digit demonstrate significantly reduced flow, suggesting a steal phenomenon from the digit by the hemodialysis access. (B) PPG waveforms of the same finger with manual compression of the hemodialysis access graft, showing return of normal flow and perfusion to the digit and confirming the steal phenomenon from the digit by the hemodialysis access. Note 1: A duplex ultrasound of the radial or ulnar artery may have been useful to demonstrate oscillating flow or reversed flow with the fully functioning graft. Note 2: An Allen's test prior to the completion of the hemodialysis access graft may have demonstrated the dominance of one of the forearm arteries over the other and/or suspicion for future compromise.

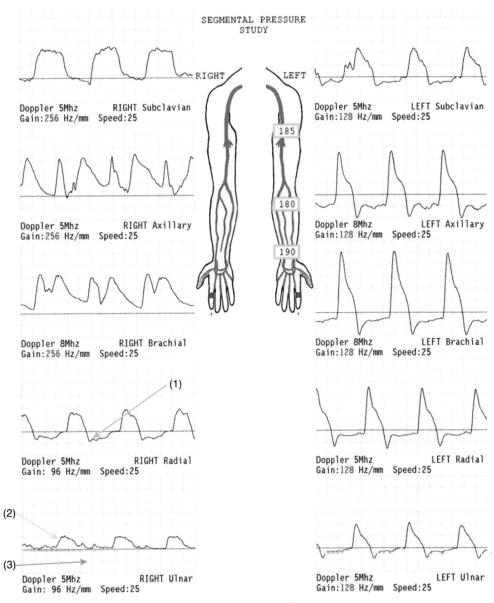

FIGURE 3.28. CW Doppler on same patient as described in Figures 3.26 and 3.27, with right arm claudication and digit ischemia from steal from hemodialysis access. Interpretation: First, CW Doppler at the level of the subclavian, axillary, and brachial arteries of the right arm demonstrates turbulent flow and loss of triphasic appearance (due to the presence of a hemodialysis access graft in that arm primarily). By themselves these waveforms could not completely exclude stenosis at the inflow. However, the PVR did not indicate compromise (see Fig. 3.26). Second, the radial and ulnar arteries resume more typical CW waveforms (without turbulence because they are distal to the dialysis access graft in this case), although demonstrating diminished flow at the ulnar artery, with: (1) delay in systole and (2) loss of triphasicity. The flow reversal (3) is probably from an adjacent vein. Normal triphasic CW Doppler waveforms were found in all arteries examined in the left arm.

CHAPTER 3

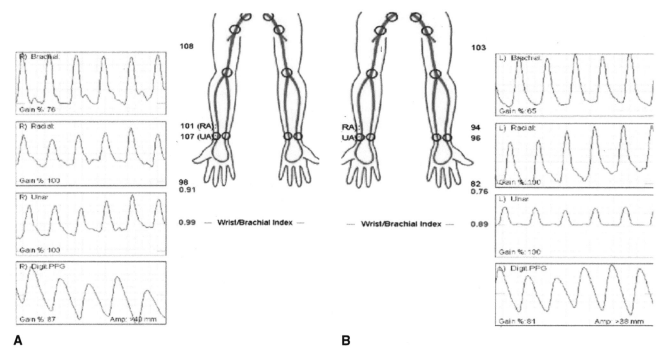

FIGURE 3.29. Difficult interpretation. Abnormal CW waveforms without compromise of flow to the digits. The CW waveforms at the level of the right and left brachial, radial, and ulnar arteries appear abnormal because the signals do not demonstrate the typical triphasic characteristics expected in a high-resistance system. However, PPG waveforms do not demonstrate decreased perfusion to the finger (normal PPG waveforms). In addition, the pressures recorded do not demonstrate significant decrease and thus compromise to perfusion. In this case, the loss of triphasic characteristics in the CW waveforms could be explained by improper technique, or it may reflect vasodilation of the distal vessels, which thus decreases the peripheral tissue resistance (not unusual, particularly in the upper extremities). Complete interpretation of this case would, however, require medical history background, as well as pulsed volume recording waveforms. Both may trigger the need for additional testing.

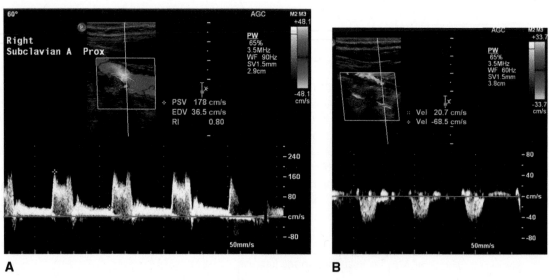

FIGURE 3.30. Subclavian artery stenosis leading to steal from the vertebral artery for perfusion of the upper extremity. Turbulence, increased velocities, and loss of waveform characteristics suggest a probable hemodynamically significant stenosis (probably more proximal from the point represented here). When significant stenosis is suspected or demonstrated in the subclavian artery, it is always good practice to examine the ipsilateral vertebral artery. As seen in this case, the significance of the stenosis is demonstrated by complete reverse flow in the ipsilateral vertebral artery demonstrating a steal of flow from the cerebral posterior circulation to the upper extremity.

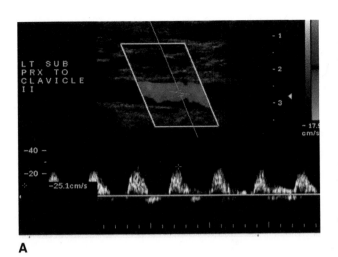

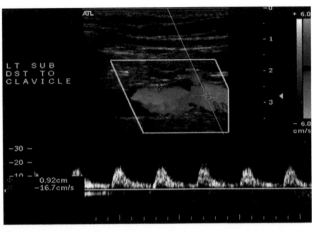

A   **B**

FIGURE 3.31.   Low velocities and progressive loss of phasicity in the subclavian artery. In this case, the low flow velocities and the progressive loss of triphasic characteristics in the pulsed wave Doppler waveforms, without any demonstrated turbulence and or visible narrowing in the vessel, suggest more proximal stenosis or even probably a more central problem at the level of the aortic (heart) valve. Examining the cerebrovascular flow in this case would be good practice, in addition, of course, to a thorough medical history.

Concluding Tips

The upper extremity arterial system, when limited to the arm and forearm, is relatively spared from diseases. Buerger's disease (despite the worldwide distribution of smoking among young adults), Takayasu's disease, and even Raynaud's disease are all relatively rare. Therefore, problems of the arterial circulation of the upper extremities will be mostly linked to arterial inflow problems at the level of the brachiocephalic trunk (on the right) and subclavian and/or axillary arteries on the right and left (although the left upper extremity seems to have a higher incidence of problems). Therefore, it is very important that the inflow be included in the examination of the etiology or cause of symptoms. Finally and as always, a good medical history will be an important part of the examination and interpretation. Hemodialysis access will be discussed further in Chapter 4.

PART TWO: UPPER EXTREMITIES

Testing the Venous Circulation

Chapter Outline

CHAPTER 4

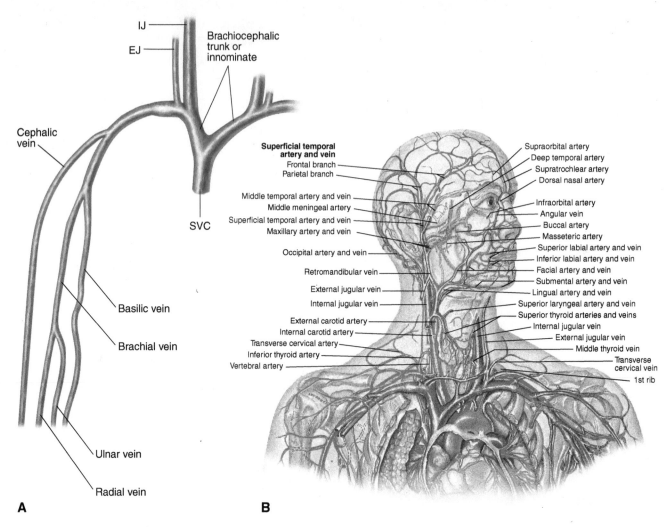

A

B

FIGURE 4.1.   Diagram of the upper extremity venous system.

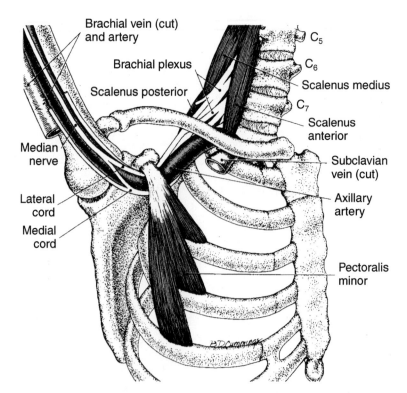

FIGURE 4.2.   Representation of the phenomenon leading to compression and thrombosis of the subclavian vein at the thoracic outlet, which is seen in Paget-Schroetter syndrome or effort thrombosis.

General Concepts in Upper Extremity Venous Evaluation

- The upper extremity is anatomically split into three portions: the hands (most distal), the forearm (between the wrist and elbow/antecubital fossa), and the arm (between the elbow and shoulder).
- The upper extremity venous system is a complex system of interconnected superficial and deep veins with frequent anatomic variations.
  - The superficial dorsal venous network of the hands will form the cephalic (on the radial side) and basilic (on the ulnar side) veins. Both cephalic and basilic veins are considered superficial veins. They are not paired and are not associated with an artery.
  - Both cephalic and basilic veins will slightly course in the ventral aspect of the forearm. The cephalic vein will assume a lateral ascending course in the arm, before draining into the proximal portion of the axillary vein. The basilic vein will course along the medial aspect of the arm and drain into the brachial vein at various levels.
  - The median cubital vein and other accessory veins usually join the cephalic and basilic veins in the forearms.
  - The superficial palmar venous network of the hands will form the radial and ulnar veins. These veins are paired alongside the arteries of the same name and are considered deep veins. These veins join usually at the level of the antecubital fossa/elbow level to form the brachial veins (also paired). Once joined by the basilic vein, the brachial veins become a single axillary vein and then a single subclavian vein at the level of the outer border of the first rib. Past the confluence with the jugular vein, the subclavian becomes the innominate vein (right and left), which drain into the superior vena cava.
  - Veins of the upper extremities have valves, although less numerous than in the lower extremities. Most valves are located proximal to confluences of veins (i.e., in the axillary vein proximal to the junction with the cephalic vein, or in the subclavian vein proximal to the junction with the external jugular vein).
- The hemodynamics of the venous flow return from the upper extremities, in contrast with the lower extremities, is strongly dependent on the heart and therefore pressure gradient. There is little to no contribution of a muscle pump (role played by the calf muscles in the lower extremities).
- The pathology of the venous system of the upper extremity is most noticeable and clinically important for thrombosis of the major draining vessels such as the axillary, subclavian, and innominate veins.
- The etiology of thrombosis in the venous system of the upper extremity is often linked to external compression (such as Paget-Schroetter syndrome, also known as spontaneous or effort thrombosis, or venous thrombosis at the thoracic outlet) or iatrogenic factors (such as insertion of wires, such as from a pacemaker, or catheters/lines, such as peripherally inserted central catheter [PICC] lines).

■ Congenital narrowing of the subclavian vein and thrombosis due to hypercoagulability syndromes or tumors are relatively rare pathologies.

■ Only approximately 2% of documented deep venous thrombosis (DVT) occurring in human arose in the upper extremities.

■ The incidence of pulmonary embolism from upper extremity DVT varies tremendously in the literature from 1–3% to 9–11%.

Tips/Rationale

■ Know the patient's medical history and occupational background.

  • Paget-Schroetter syndrome, or its less severe form known as McLeery's syndrome (intermittent compression at the thoracic outlet with symptoms but no thrombosis), are most often seen in very active, young, and otherwise healthy patients. Competitive athletes and workers using repetitive, forceful motions of the upper body and arms will be the most prone to these syndromes.

  • Central, acute thrombosis requires immediate and aggressive treatment through thrombectomy or, more widely accepted, through catherter-directed thrombolysis.

■ Know the rationale for the test.

  • The venous system of the upper extremity should be thoroughly evaluated before hemodialysis access creation or placement.

  • The size of the veins that could be used for the graft would be important, but the condition of the venous drainage would be crucial.

  • Superficial veins may also be harvested for lower extremity bypass graft and/or coronary bypass graft.

■ Note: The postevaluation of hemodialysis access will be covered in a separate chapter.

Protocol Algorithm

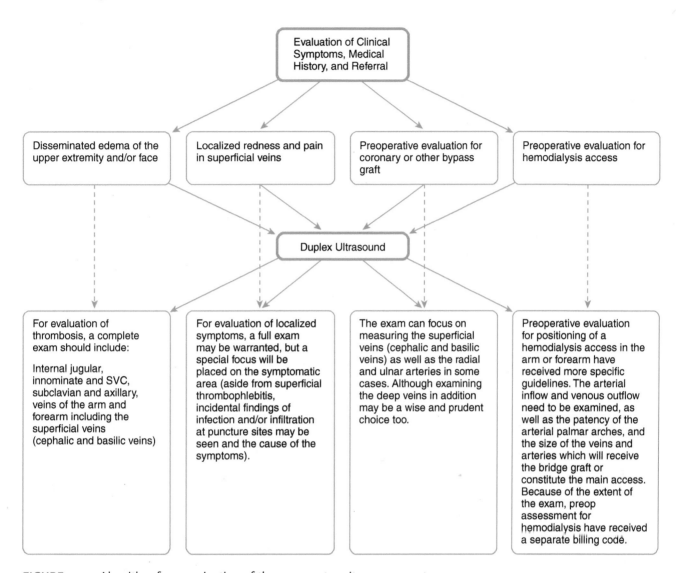

FIGURE 4.3. Algorithm for examination of the upper extremity venous system.

Duplex Exam of Upper Extremity Venous Circulation

Test Preparation

- The test preparation's main challenge is ensuring that the patient's position is conducive to the best visibility of the vessels and comfortable for the patient and sonographer. The patient may be supine or sitting.

- The particular situation surrounding the request for the test will often dictate the most appropriate equipment setting and positioning.

- The examination should preferably be bilateral, particularly if effort thrombosis or Paget-Schroetter syndrome is suspected. The problem has been reported to be bilateral in 60% of cases with or without apparent symptoms at the time of the examination.

- Preoperative evaluation for hemodialysis access graft is also recommended to be performed bilaterally. The rationale here is that even when the surgery is well planned and the patient and physician have elected to place the access in the nondominant arm, evaluating the other arm may save time. An inadvertent placement of an intravenous (IV) line in the arm to receive the access may trigger a change of plan at the last minute.

Testing Sequence

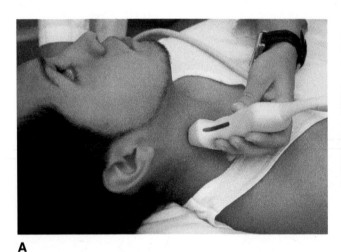
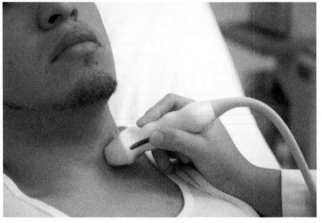

A   **B**

FIGURE 4.4.   Start (or end) the exam by visualizing and evaluating the internal jugular vein (IJV). It may be valuable to visualize the portion of the internal jugular vein located at the junction with the innominate, the innominate vein, and the superior vena cava. These veins are difficult to access by duplex ultrasound. Using a transducer with a smaller footprint (such as a phased array) with a lower frequency, placed in the suprasternal notch may offer an adequate technique and window.

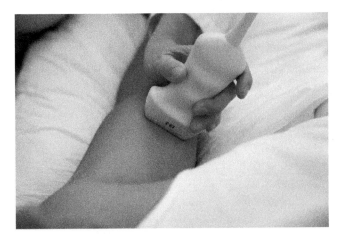

FIGURE 4.5.   Arm resting on a pillow or arm rest if available can help the patient maintain an adequate position for evaluation of the arteries or veins, here for transverse views.

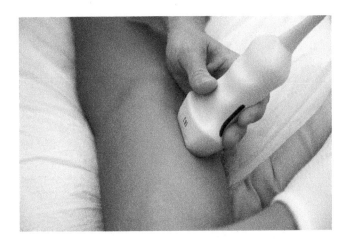

FIGURE 4.6.   Arm resting on a pillow or arm rest if available can help the patient maintain an adequate position for evaluation of the arteries or veins, here for longitudinal views.

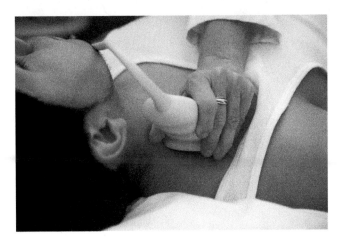

FIGURE 4.7.   This position allows for the examination of the subclavian artery and vein (useful for a pre-operative evaluation for hemodialysis access) as well as for following the vessels toward the arm in a longitudinal approach.

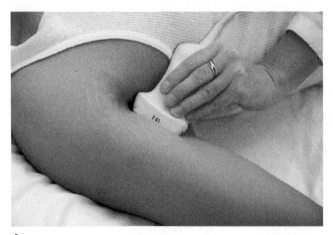

A

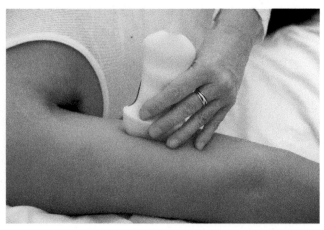

B

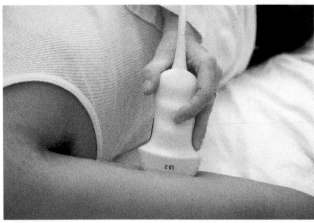

C

FIGURE 4.8.   These positions allow for viewing the veins and arteries (useful when performing a pre-operative exam for future placement of a hemodialysis access) in longitudinal, and evaluating the flow physiology by PW and/or color Doppler. (A) Evaluation of the distal axillary, proximal brachial. (B) Evaluation of the brachial and basilic. (C) Evaluation of the distal brachial and basilic, as well as confluence of radial and ulnar.

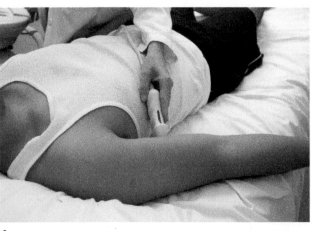

A

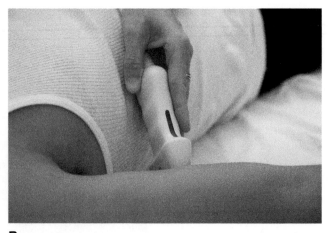

B

FIGURE 4.9.   These positions allow for viewing the major deep veins and the basilic vein in transverse to perform compression and exclude thrombosis. (Continued)

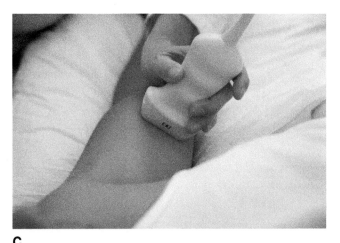

C

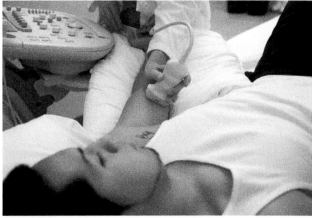

D

FIGURE 4.9. (Continued)

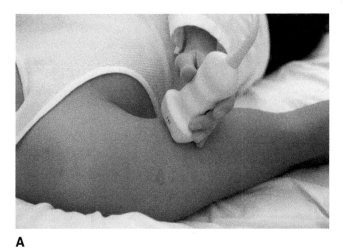

A

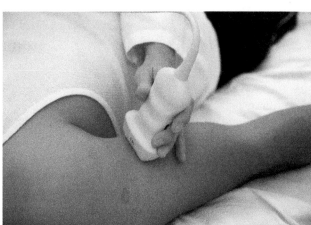

B

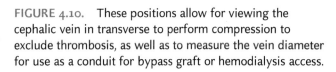

C

FIGURE 4.10. These positions allow for viewing the cephalic vein in transverse to perform compression to exclude thrombosis, as well as to measure the vein diameter for use as a conduit for bypass graft or hemodialysis access.

Results and Interpretation

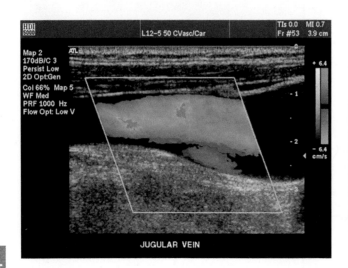

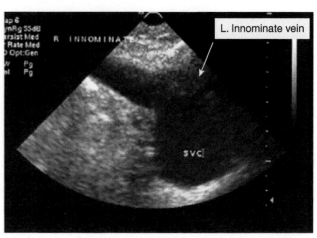

FIGURE 4.11.   Evaluation of the IJV could be done by compression (just like most other accessible veins). However, thrombosis of the jugular vein often results from indwelling catheter or other lines and compression may not be very comfortable for the patient or even possible (due to surgical dressing, edema, etc.). Evaluating the IJV for patency with color Doppler in transverse and/or longitudinal views is an alternative to compression. Color should fill the entire lumen.

FIGURE 4.12.   Suprasternal approach for visualization of the superior vena cava (SVC). Vein compression at this level is not possible to exclude thrombosis. Other techniques such as color Doppler, power Doppler, or pulse Doppler, in addition to visualization in gray scale, should be used to evaluate the presence or absence of thrombus (always correlating observations to history).

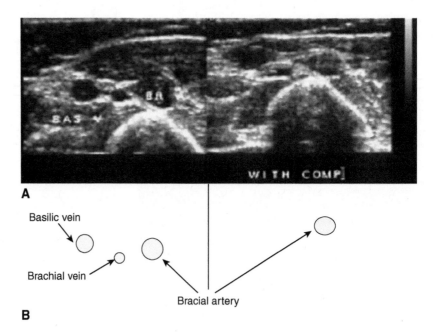

FIGURE 4.13.   Example of evaluation of patency of upper extremity veins with guided compression. Normal compression of the basilic and brachial veins with the ultrasound transducer excludes the presence of thrombosis.

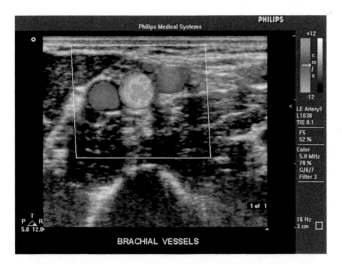

FIGURE 4.14. Evaluation of veins patency in transverse using color Doppler. Here both brachial veins (arrows) are patent (evident by complete color fill of the vessels).

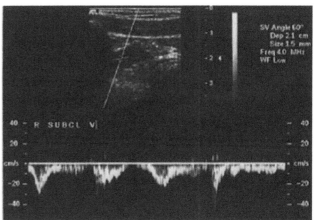

FIGURE 4.15. Proximal subclavian vein with typical slightly pulsatile but phasic pulsed wave Doppler waveforms. The pulsatility is due to the closeness of the heart; the phasicity corresponds to the phases of respiration and the changes of pressure in the thoracic cavity that increase (during inspiration) or decrease/stop (during expiration) the venous return from the upper extremities and head. The subclavian vein and part of the axillary vein in most individuals are not amenable to ultrasound-guided compression to evaluate for the presence or absence of thrombosis. As cited earlier, color Doppler, power Doppler, and pulse Doppler are the techniques used for such evaluation.

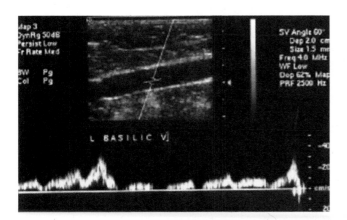

FIGURE 4.16. Another typical example of pulse Doppler waveforms in a vein of the upper extremity. Here the basilic vein displays pulsatile and phasic flow.

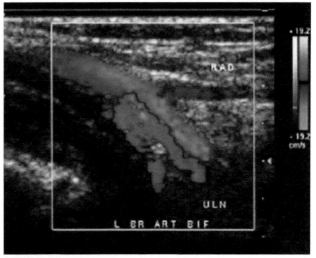

FIGURE 4.17. Longitudinal view of the brachial bifurcation with arteries and veins. Evaluation of the veins in a longitudinal view would allow for understanding the anatomic and relative positions of the artery and veins. Adding color or pulse Doppler will allow for assessment of flow pattern and direction.

CHAPTER 4

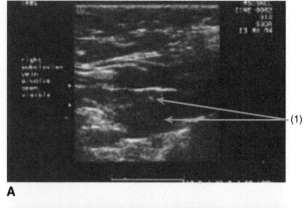

A

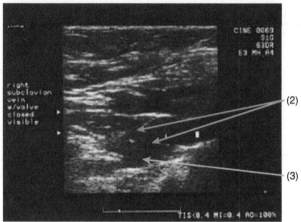

B

FIGURE 4.18.   Depiction of valve closure in the proximal subclavian vein. Valves in the upper body are less numerous than in the lower extremity veins. (1) Subclavian vein with open valve leaflets. (2) Subclavian vein with valves closed. (3) The rouleaux effects proximal to the closed valve show that the valve is completely closed.

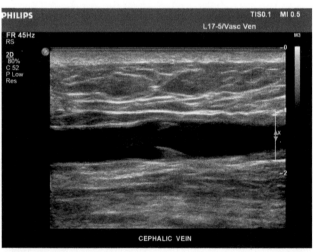

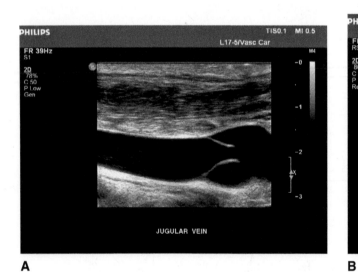

A

B

FIGURE 4.19.   Valves of the internal jugular vein and cephalic vein. Courtesy of Philips.

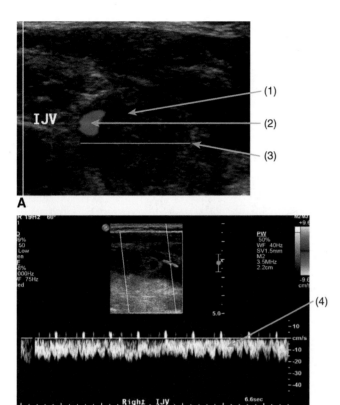

A

B

FIGURE 4.20.   Sample of thrombosis in the internal jugular vein with either recanalization or non–completely occluding thrombus. Partial thrombus in an internal jugular vein in grayscale (1). Note: Depending on the age of the thrombus it may be difficult to evaluate the extent of the thrombus in B-mode alone. Partial thrombus in the internal jugular vein (2) with some flow (3) and the diameter of the vessel. Note that the pulsed wave Doppler waveform shows continuous (yet still slightly pulsatile) flow around the thrombus (4), which may indicate a more proximal extension of the thrombus to the brachiocephalic vein and/or superior vena cava (SVC). If Dopplers of both internal jugular veins are similar, the the thrombus probably involves the SVC.

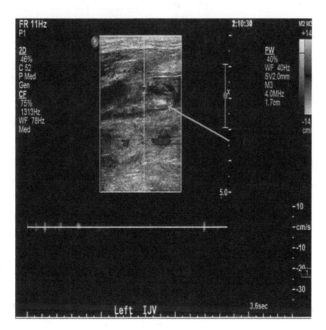

FIGURE 4.21.   Complete thrombosis of the internal jugular vein seen by mixed echogenic materials (arrow) within the vessel lumen but also by absence of color on color Doppler and absence of signal on PW Doppler.

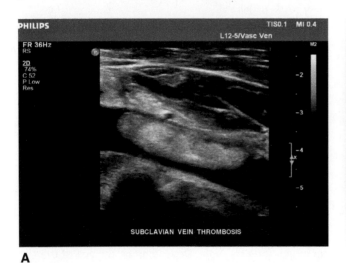

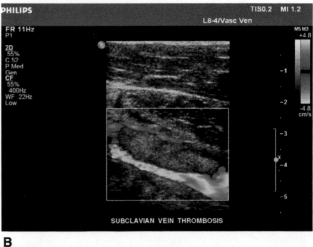

A

B

FIGURE 4.22.   Thrombosis in the subclavian vein. Courtesy of Philips.

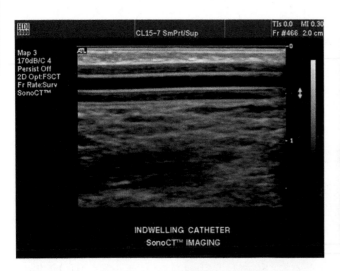

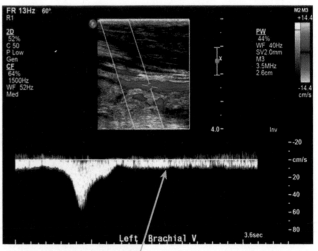

FIGURE 4.23.   Vein with indwelling catheter but no evidence of thrombosis. However the vein should also be examined in a transverse view to perform ultrasound guided compression and exclude the presence of anechoic thrombus with color or power Doppler to demonstrate flow around the catheter. Courtesy of Philips.

FIGURE 4.24.   Another sample of pulse Doppler waveforms in an upper extremity vein that is suspicious for more proximal thrombosis, compression, or another form of obstruction. Brachial vein with pulse Doppler shows loss of pulsatility and phasicity (arrow; i.e., continuous flow still responding to distal augmentation). This finding probably indicates thrombosis or compression of more proximal veins.

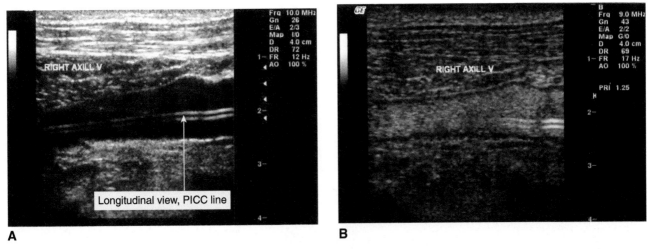

A **B**

FIGURE 4.25. Sample of a vein with a PICC line. (A) Right axillary vein with PICC line in a longitudinal view of the vein. (B) Right axillary vein with PICC line, shown here with B flow. B flow showing flow filling the lumen of the vessel around the catheter excludes here the presence of thrombus.

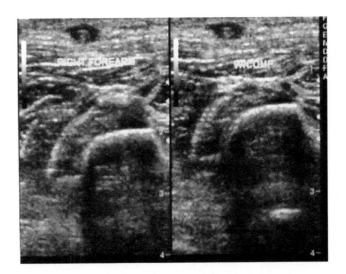

FIGURE 4.26. Superficial vein in the right forearm with a line present in the lumen. Manual compression with the transducer was performed to evaluate for the presence or absence of thrombus around the line. The vein does not compress completely around the line in this picture, suggesting acute thrombosis around the line. Confirmation with color or power Doppler should be performed.

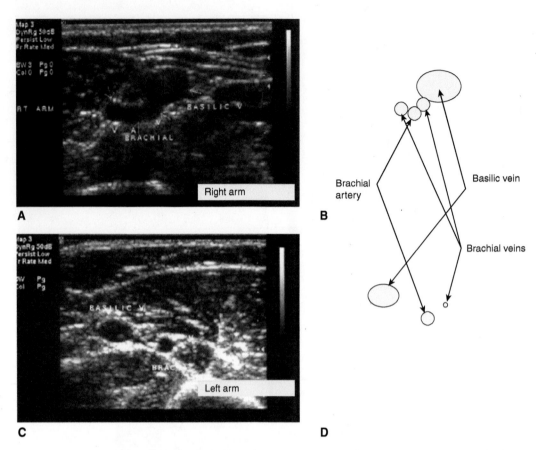

FIGURE 4.27. View and position of the basilic vein in the upper arm. The basilic vein is medial to the brachial artery and veins. It can be used for bypass or dialysis access.

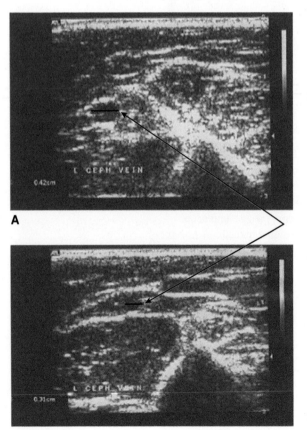

FIGURE 4.28. Sample of measurements of the cephalic vein (arrows) in transverse view for either a preoperative exam for a lower extremity bypass or a hemodialysis access. The measurements are: (A) 4.2 mm (or 0.42 cm) and (B) 3.1 mm (or 0.31 cm), which was taken distally.

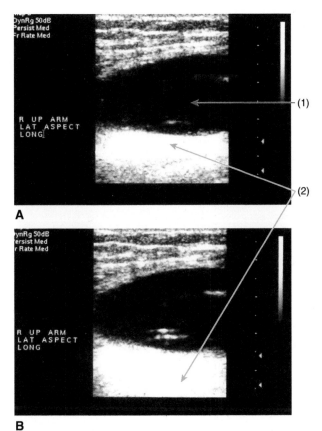

FIGURE 4.29.   Example of incidental findings when evaluating the upper extremity venous system. The patient presented with redness and swelling at the site investigated. (1) Lateral aspect of the arm. A large fluid collection is noted in the symptomatic area. This could represent infiltration from an IV or an inflammation of infection in the subcutaneous tissue. (2) Note also the posterior enhancement due to the acoustic window created by the fluid collection.

CHAPTER 4

Concluding Tips

Upper extremity venous evaluation can be a challenging exam because most large draining veins are difficult to access and assess with conventional methods for evaluation of the main pathology of veins (i.e., thrombosis). Indeed because of their anatomic positions, the innominate, subclavian, and most of the axillary veins cannot be evaluated by manual compression with the ultrasound transducer. Thoroughly examining the flow patterns with pulse Doppler, but also color and/or power Doppler, will provide invaluable information and can confirm clinical suspicion. Unless the symptoms are localized, it will always be good practice to evaluate both upper extremities and the draining system as close as possible to the most central vein—the superior vena cava (SVC). The following section will cover the evaluation of hemodialysis access.

General Concepts in Examining Hemodialysis Access

This section will be slightly different in concept and scope than most others in this manual. This section will cover the use of ultrasound technology for the examination of a treatment procedure created not to relieve vascular problems but to supplement or replace the functions of a failing organ. In this case, the failing organs are the kidneys, and the treatment procedure is the creation of a hemodialysis access. The basic idea is to create a conduit with a high volume of blood that can be filtered through an external and artificial kidney, therefore replacing the daily filtration normally occurring through the kidneys.

- Hemodialysis is one of the methods (with peritoneal dialysis) used to replace one of the important functions of the kidneys (i.e., the continuous filtration of blood to remove electrolytes and other waste metabolites).
- Dialysis is usually required when the kidneys have lost approximately 90% of their function.
- Several conditions, such as diabetes, hypertension, and inflammation of the filtration system of the kidneys or small vessels within the kidneys, can cause the kidneys to fail. However, diabetes is the leading cause of kidney failure, followed closely by hypertension.
- Hemodialysis requires the creation of a conduit within the body for:
  - Easy access, so the technicians can easily find the conduit and the patient can be comfortably connected to the dialyzer for several hours
  - High volume of blood to be delivered and thus filtered within a few hours (and usually every other day)
  - For the former point, the most common sites are the wrist or forearm.
  - For the latter point, the best solution is to connect an artery to a vein, either directly or through the interposition of a synthetic graft.
- Arteriovenous fistula (AVF) is used when the access is a direct connection between the artery and vein, and looped graft or graft is used when the connection involves the interposition of a synthetic graft.
- Connecting a high-pressure system (the artery) to a low-pressure system (the vein) will force the blood to be rerouted toward the vein and thus raise the volume of blood through that conduit. Although the effect is immediate once the connection between the artery and vein is done, using the conduit for dialysis purposes requires some time for what is called "maturation." This process of maturation includes:
  - A vein conduit that has sufficiently dilated (ideally to ≥ 0.5 cm in diameter) to accommodate the cannula used with the dialyzer
  - An adequate volume of flow (at least > 350 mL/min and ideally around 400–500 mL/min)
  - A matured conduit of approximately 10 cm long in the draining vein for optimal rotation of puncture site
- AVFs usually require a longer time to mature than looped grafts.

Tips/Rationale

- Despite an increase in the incidence and use of hemodialysis, reimbursement for evaluation does not include (as of 2008) regular follow-up, as it does with bypass grafts.

- Request for assessment of function of dialysis accesses (and reimbursement) needs to be based on signs of clinical dysfunction or indications, such as:

  - Loss or decreased strength of thrill felt over the access. The thrill, which is palpable over the access on a normally functioning access, is due to the high-flow volume

  - Problems with cannulation, circulation time, or flow volume rate found at the time of dialysis

  - Long maturation time after the surgical procedure

  - Edema of the extremity housing the access

  - Suspicion of pseudoaneurysm or aneurysm

  - Pain in the hands or fingers during or after dialysis or ulceration of the fingers

- Before undertaking ultrasound assessment, it is crucial that:

  - The sonographer obtains a detailed description of the type of access performed

  - The sonographer obtains a detailed description of the signs and symptoms prompting the request for evaluation. The rationale for this point will be discussed in the Testing Sequence and/or Results and Interpretation sections.

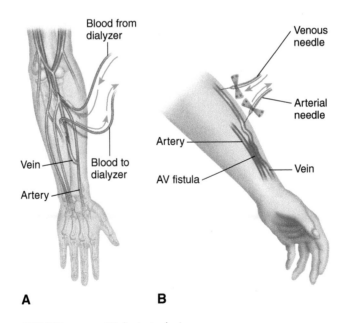

A   **B**

FIGURE 4.30.   Dialysis technique.

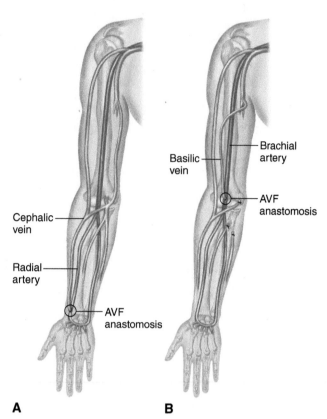

Cephalic
vein

Radial
artery

AVF
anastomosis

A

Basilic
vein

Brachial
artery

AVF
anastomosis

B

FIGURE 4.31.   Common configuration of hemodialysis accesses using veins. (A) Also known as Brescia-Cimino fistula. (B) Usually referred to as transposed basilic vein fistula.

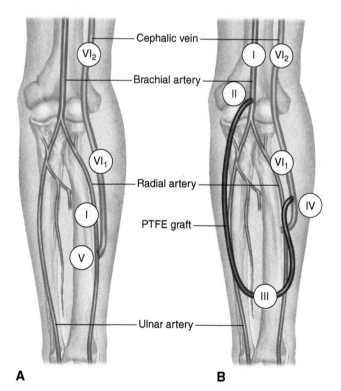

Cephalic vein

Brachial artery

Radial artery

PTFE graft

Ulnar artery

A

B

FIGURE 4.32.   Most common configuration of hemodialysis access with synthetic material. As with arterial bypass grafts, the name used to refer to the access usually is composed of the inflow artery, outflow vein, and type of graft used. Shown here is a brachial artery to basilic vein loop graft.

Protocol Algorithm

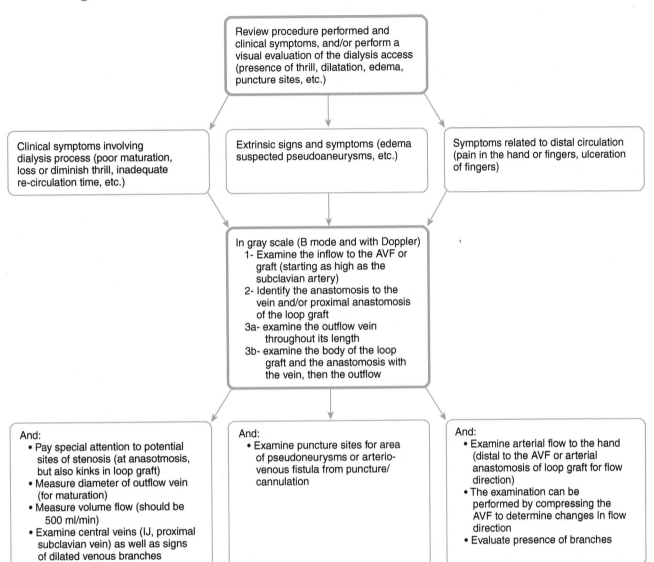

FIGURE 4.33.   Examination algorithm. Algorithm based on information provided by the Society for Vascular Ultrasound (Vascular Professional Guidelines) and the American Institute of Ultrasound in Medicine (Practice Guideline).

Duplex Exam for Examining Hemodialysis Access

Test Preparation and Hand Test Sequence

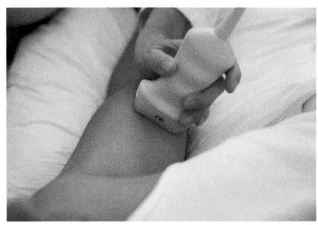

A

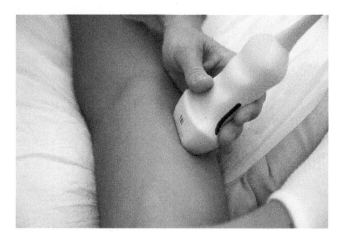

B

FIGURE 4.34.   Patient's arm is comfortably resting on a pillow.

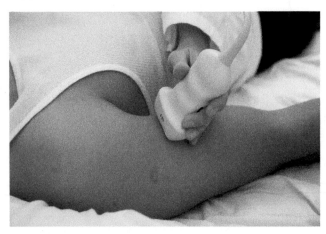

A

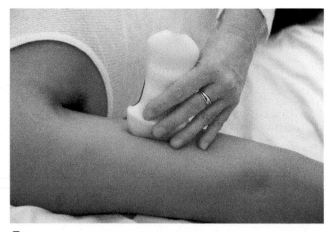

B

FIGURE 4.35.   The dialysis access, whether AVF or loop graft, should include all sections outlined in the protocol algorithm (Fig. 4.33). Views can alternate between transverse and longitudinal as seen here to obtain the data. The scanning approach will vary based on the position of the access. It is therefore important if not crucial to obtain operative notes to understand the position of the access.

Results and Interpretation

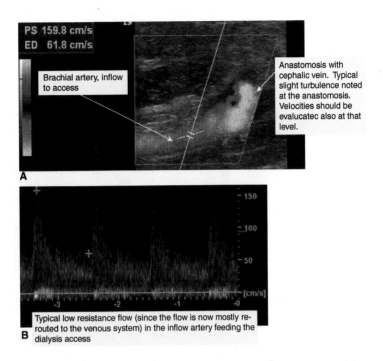

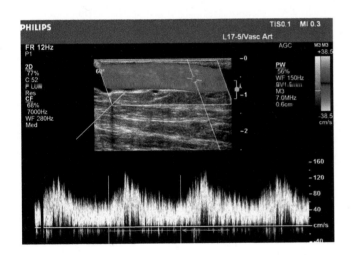

FIGURE 4.36. Sample of evaluation of a matured dialysis access created between the brachial artery and cephalic vein. The waveform is taken at the brachial artery proximal to the access (site I on diagram in Fig. 4.32).

FIGURE 4.37. Measuring flow volume. Note: This feature is available in calculation package on most equipment; when it is not, the calculation can be done manually as long as the ultrasound equipment has a feature to calculate mean flow velocities through one cardiac cycle. To measure the flow volume (or volume flow), (1) measure diameter of the conduit (calculate the surface area = π × radius squared). (2) Obtain mean flow velocities throughout one cardiac cycle with a Doppler sample volume set to the diameter of the vessel. Volume flow = surface area × mean velocities (unit will be cm³/s), then multiply by 60 to get units in milliliters per minutes. Courtesy of Philips.

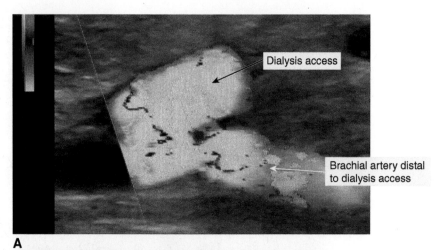

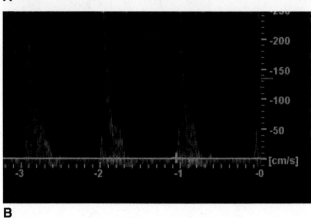

FIGURE 4.38.   AVF between brachial artery and cephalic vein, with the Doppler sample taken in the brachial artery distal to the dialysis access. High-resistance flow should be noted (and resumed) in the artery distal to the AVF or loop graft take off, since that flow now feeds the distal territories in the forearm, hand, and fingers. The direction of flow should be directed toward these territories. When or if the flow appears reversed and the symptoms correlate with lack of flow to the territories distal to the AVF or loop graft, a steal phenomenon from the forearm by the dialysis access should be suspected. To confirm, the AVF or venous outflow from loop graft could be manually compressed (shut down) while the artery distal to the graft is evaluated by Doppler; a change of flow direction (to normal direction) should be observed.

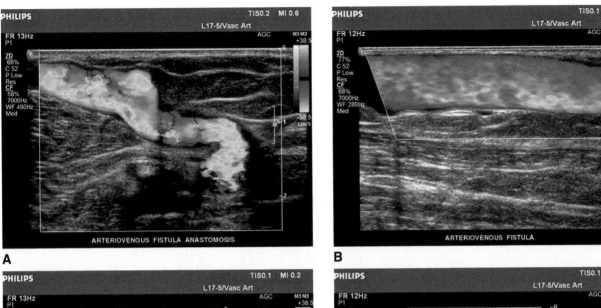

A

B

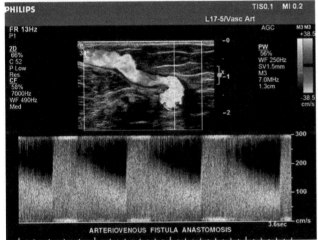

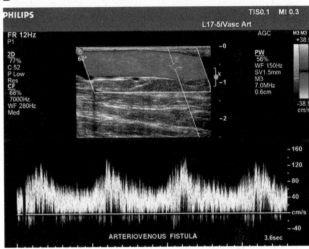

C

FIGURE 4.39.   AVF between brachial artery and cephalic vein, with the Doppler sample taken in the proximal aspect of the dialysis access (site VI1 on diagram in Fig. 4.32). Assess velocities, structural changes (dilatation, pseudoaneurysms), and sites of narrowing are seen throughout the conduit and at anastomoses. Caution: There is no recorded consensus on truly acceptable velocities within a dialysis access (although velocities < 100 cm/s are suspicious of poor function or poor maturity), but know that velocities will normally increase within a well-functioning access with maturity of the access. It is not unusual to have increased flow velocities at the anastomoses, particularly with synthetic graft, due to kinking of the graft. Clinical signs and symptoms should be strictly considered with these results before revision is undertaken. Criteria for stenosis usually follow the rule for bypass grafts and peripheral arteries, such as a doubling of velocity from a more proximal and nondiseased segment suggests 50% stenosis and a tripling of velocity suggests a 75% stenosis. Courtesy of Philips.

CHAPTER 4

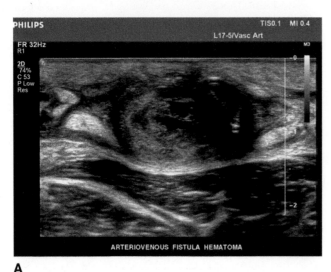

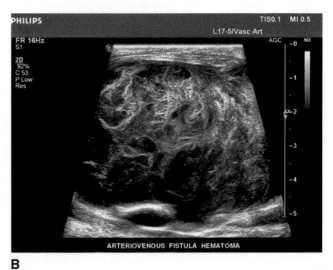

A

B

FIGURE 4.40. Hematoma in arteriovenous fistula (dialysis access). Courtesy of Philips.

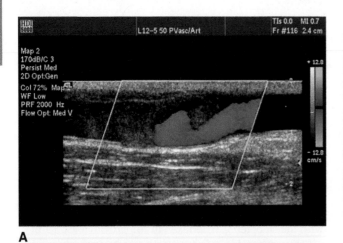

A

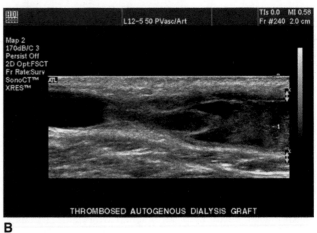

B

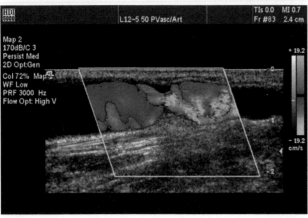

C

FIGURE 4.41. Complications in autogenous dialysis access: (A) narrowing of a part of the vein graft, (B) stenosis often followed by decreased flow velocities and turbulence leading to thrombosis, and (C) slow flow itself (from multiple causes) can lead to thrombosis of the access.

Concluding Tips

Evaluation of dialysis accesses is a challenging exam. More than ever, a thorough understanding of basic hemodynamics and flow direction is needed, along with an open mind and critical thinking to anticipate and understand the changes in anatomy and, most importantly, physiology that the creation of the access will trigger. Communication with the surgeon who created the access, the dialysis center that treats the patient on a regular basis, and the patient (or caregiver) is also crucial for a successful and meaningful evaluation of this treatment option. Finally, and as for many if not all other exams in the vascular laboratory, the examination of a dialysis access should be tackled as a new challenge each time, even on returning patients. The vascular system is truly a dynamic system, and one should always consider every piece of information available as an integral part of the exam, every time.

CHAPTER 5

PART THREE: ABDOMEN

Testing the Abdominal Aorta

Chapter Outline

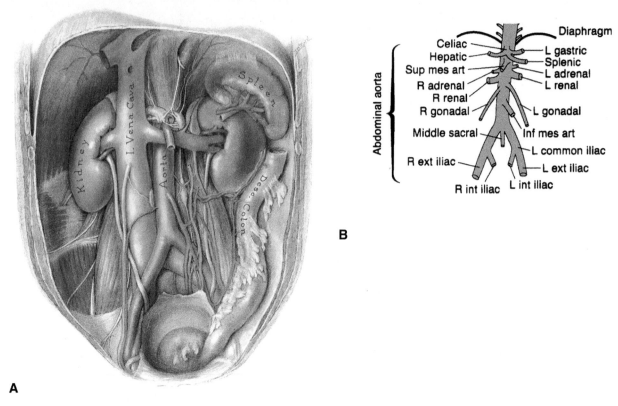

Diaphragm
Celiac
Hepatic
Sup mes art
R adrenal
R renal
R gonadal
Middle sacral
R ext iliac
R int iliac

L gastric
Splenic
L adrenal
L renal
L gonadal
Inf mes art
L common iliac
L ext iliac
L int iliac

Abdominal aorta

Kidney
I. Vena Cava
Aorta
Spleen
Desc. Colon

A

B

FIGURE 5.1. Diagrams of the vasculature of the abdomen with organs.

General Concepts in Abdominal Aorta Evaluation

Duplex ultrasound is a reliable, convenient, and safe technology for screening, evaluating disease progression, and following-up on treatment procedures for one of the main pathologies of the abdominal aorta, aneurysm, or aneurismal dilatation. This does not imply that the abdominal aorta's sole pathology is aneurismal disease. Indeed, as an artery, the aorta is also prone to occlusive diseases through atherosclerotic or thrombotic processes. In addition, the etiology and progressive course of aneurismal disease are either associated with or trigger other problems affecting this particular vessel and the vessels branching from it. Finally, the treatments or procedures used or performed on the abdominal aorta or its branches may also have unwanted or unforeseen consequences on this artery.

The overall goal of this chapter is to provide an overview of the tips and techniques for the evaluation of the abdominal aorta by duplex ultrasound. The results and interpretations will focus on aneurysms because of its predominance regarding referrals to vascular laboratories for abdominal aorta evaluation.

Tips/Rationale

Rationale: Why focus on aneurysms?

- While occlusive diseases of the aorta are not uncommon (or at least not less common than aneurysms), the patients with such suspected condition will usually be referred for claudication symptoms and therefore evaluation of the lower extremities' arterial system. Findings of aortic occlusive disease will usually be based on the results of a physiologic study and could lead to performing a duplex ultrasound of the abdominal aorta or other imaging modalities.

- Several large and smaller epidemiologic studies over the past decade have in some sense (since it may not have been the primary reason for the study) uncovered that abdominal aortic aneurysm may have been for a long time an under-diagnosed condition and the cause of death in more cases than previously thought.

- These epidemiologic studies and others, as well as the work of several physicians, have resulted in the enactment of the Screening for Abdominal Aortic Aneurysm Very Efficiently (SAAAVE) Act. Since January of 2007, through this act, males over 65 and a history of smoking, and males/females with a family history of aortic aneurysms can undergo a screening evaluation for aortic aneurysm as part of their first *Welcome to Medicare* physical exam.

- In addition studies also often lead to new discovery, or new theory about risk factors and pathological processes. This holds true for aneurysms of the abdominal aorta.

- Finally, the development of endovascular repair or treatment of abdominal aortic aneurysms has gained a tremendous and widespread acceptance. The prevention of the deadliest consequence of aneurismal disease, rupture followed by massive hemorrhaging, can now be undertaken more safely.

Tips:

- Duplex examination of the abdominal aorta can be challenging because of the anatomic location of the vessel, which, on an anterior approach, is behind the intestines and, on a posterior approach, is behind the spine. Both locations greatly limit the transmission of sound.

- However, duplex ultrasound allows for constant adjustment of the imaging/scanning approach by the operator and allows the possible evaluation of:
  - The tortuosity of the vessel,
  - And the position of pathology in regard to landmarks (such as the renal arteries, inferior mesenteric artery, and iliac arteries),
  - All with the goal to provide accurate measurements.

- The scanning approach needs to be considered when documenting measurements in the aorta (the rationale here is that some research studies have shown that the formation and progression of aneurysms are not uniformly distributed along the circumference of the vessel, AND progression in one dimension compared to the other may have an impact on the prognosis or incidence of rupture).

- A new endovascular technique to repair the abdominal aortic aneurysm (known as EVAR) has added challenges in documentation before and after the procedure, including:

  - The position of the aneurysm in relation to other vascular structures needs to be known before the procedure (particularly the distance from the take off of the renal arteries to the proximal aspect of the aneurysm)

  - The precise size and appearance (tortuosity and presence and amount of plaque or thrombosis, which may render the insertion of the endovascular graft difficult) of the aneurismal sac

  - The precise size and appearance of the aorta proximal to the aneurysm where the endograft will rest, as well as the size and appearance of the common or external iliac arteries where the distal portion of the endograft will be attached

  - The presence and precise location of branches (such as the internal iliac arteries to induce, for example, vascular impotence after EVAR)

- The previous considerations, although important for open repair and completeness of the assessment, are not as crucial because the vascular surgeon will be able to assess the situation (particularly branches) during the surgical procedure.

Protocol Algorithm

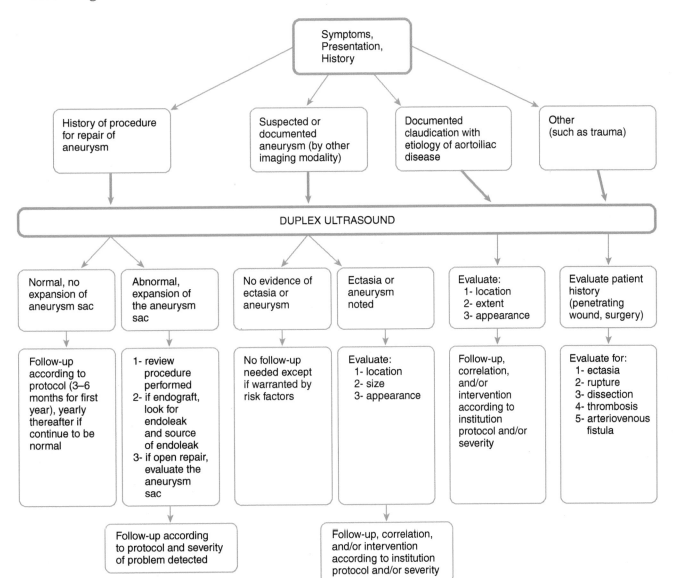

FIGURE 5.2. Algorithm for examination of the abdominal aorta.

Imaging Studies by Duplex

Test Preparation

The test preparation, aside from selecting the proper software package and transducer for abdominal ultrasound, is basically focused on ensuring the proper position and preparation of the patient for adequate imaging. It is generally accepted that the patient should be instructed to fast for at least 12 hours prior to the exam, including refraining from chewing gum or tobacco and smoking a minimum of 1 hour before the test. However, performing the exam even when the patient has not fasted is feasible and, in most cases, adequate. Patients who are required to take medications on a daily basis can do so with a glass of water or juice before the exam.

The most appropriate positions for examination of the abdominal aorta are described in the picture sequence below. Whereas having the patient supine or in a lateral decubitus position is optimal, we need to be flexible and creative and envision that, in a few extraordinary circumstances, the examination may have to be attempted with the patient sitting, with the patient's back slightly reclined.

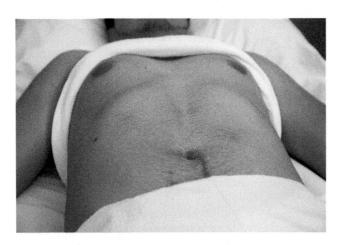

FIGURE 5.3.   Most common and versatile position for examination of the aorta and inferior vena cava (IVC).

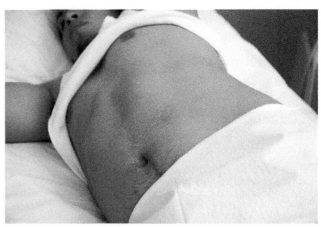

FIGURE 5.4.   Alternate position to minimize acoustic shadowing from intestine.

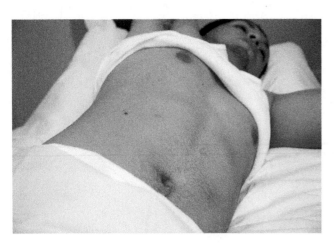

FIGURE 5.5.   Alternate position. Despite the fact that the anatomic position of the aorta is to the left of the spine, this position may be a possible alternative.

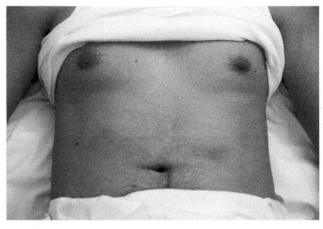

FIGURE 5.6.   Position to be used at the discretion of all involved. This position will involve many challenges but may be the only option and is thus worth trying.

Testing Sequence

Please remember that there are no right or wrong chronologic sequences per se. This tip is included to emphasize the need for flexibility in undertaking and completing the exam. It is particularly important here and for all exams involving the abdomen because, despite the best preparation possible, no one can ever control or predict how the intestinal content will affect the imaging. This means that you may have to start the exam at the level of the iliac arteries and work your way proximal to evaluate the aorta.

However, you will need to ensure that you follow the protocol prescribed in your laboratory and obtain all data and documentation. With that said, the exam should include the evaluation of the entire length of the abdominal aorta with sequential measurements proximally (usually at the level of the superior mesenteric artery), in the mid portion (usually at the level of the renal arteries), and distally (usually above the iliac bifurcation and/or the level of the inferior mesenteric artery). We will follow the testing sequence with the patient in a supine position and assume an anterior scanning approach. As discussed previously, it is possible that this approach will have to be modified under some circumstances. Refer to the section on scanning approaches and their implications to measurements of structures found in the introduction chapter for further information.

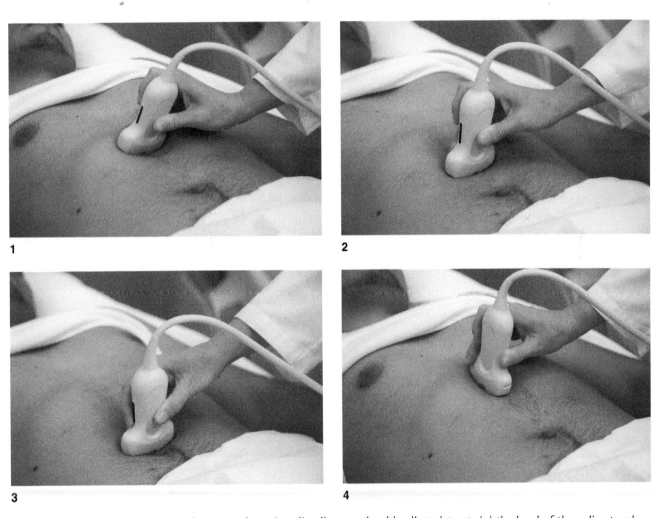

1

2

3

4

FIGURE 5.7. Starting at the diaphragm and moving distally, you should collect data at: (1) the level of the celiac trunk or superior mesenteric artery (SMA), (2) the level of the renal arteries, (3) slightly above the iliac bifurcation, and (4) for each common iliac artery.

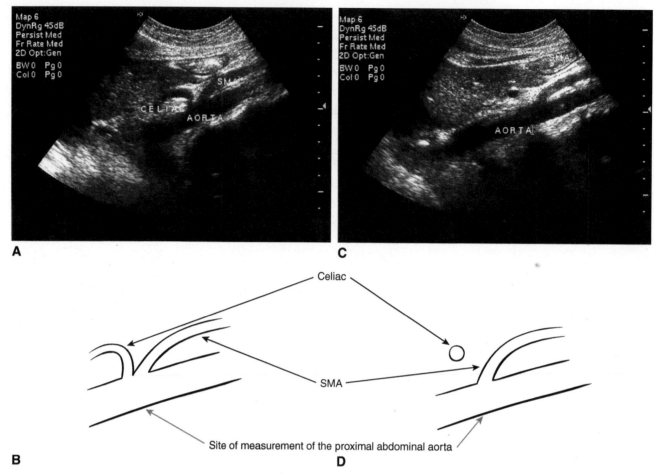

A

C

B

D

FIGURE 5.8.   Recognizing landmarks in evaluation of the abdominal aorta: celiac trunk and SMA. Site of measurement of the proximal abdominal aorta.

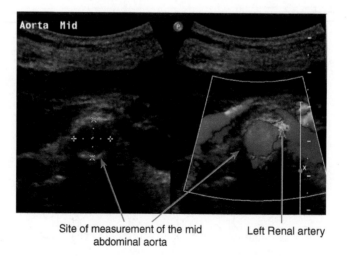

Site of measurement of the mid
abdominal aorta

Left Renal artery

FIGURE 5.9.   Recognizing landmarks in evaluation of the
abdominal aorta: renal arteries. Site of measurement of
the mid-abdominal aorta.

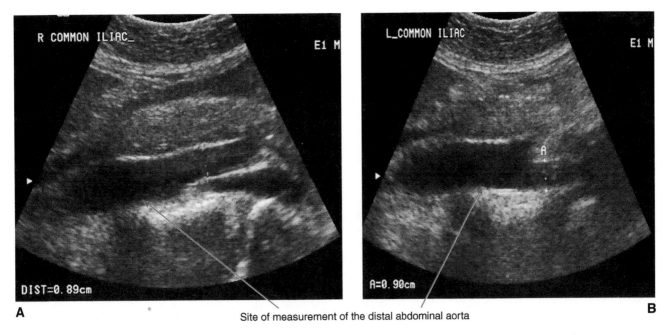

Site of measurement of the distal abdominal aorta

FIGURE 5.10. Recognizing landmarks in evaluation of the abdominal aorta: common iliac arteries. Site of measurement of the distal abdominal aorta will be 1 to 2 cm proximal to the iliac bifurcation.

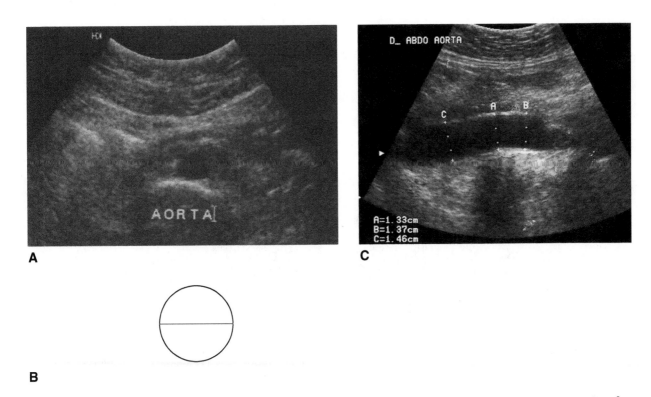

FIGURE 5.11. Techniques and meaning of measurements of the abdominal aorta. (A and B) On a transverse view from an anterior approach, the outer wall-to-outer wall measurement as depicted here will correspond to side-to-side diameter. (C) On a longitudinal view from an anterior approach, the outer wall-to-outer wall measurement as depicted here will correspond to the anteroposterior diameter.

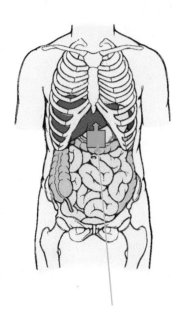

A

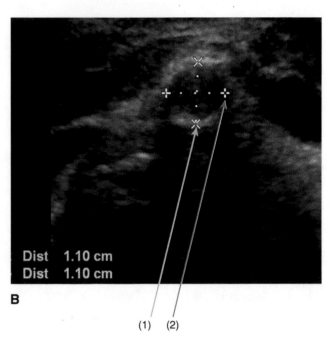

B

(1)   (2)

FIGURE 5.12.   Caution: All images are assuming anterior approach. (A) True anterior approach, transverse view. (B) Measurements obtained: (1) anteroposterior diameter and (2) lateral (side-to-side) diameter. Note: All measurements should be taken from outer wall to outer wall.

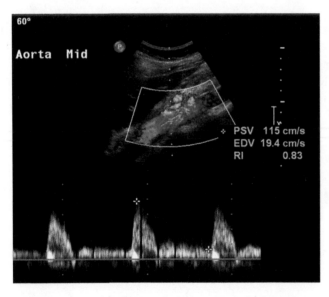

FIGURE 5.13.   It is recommended to use pulse Doppler at the sites of measurement. The same rules for Doppler evaluation apply here (i.e., Doppler angle of 60° or less, sample gate within the stream of the flow and parallel to the vessel walls).

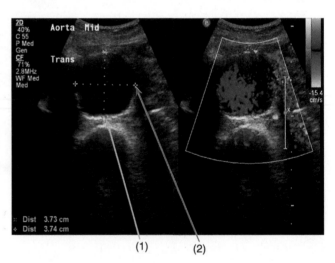

(1)   (2)

FIGURE 5.14.   Measuring the diameter of an aneurysm. Both anteroposterior (1) and lateral diameters (2) are measured in the same transverse view.

Results and Interpretation

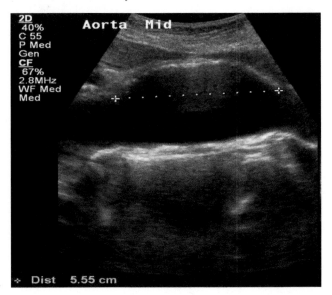

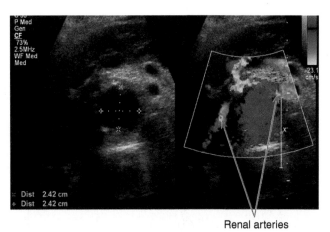

Renal arteries

FIGURE 5.15.   Measuring the length of an aneurysm in a longitudinal view. It is important here to use all the features offered by the equipment you are using (if available). Some aneurysms can span several centimeters in length. If your equipment has a panoramic feature, here is the time to use it, or else use the longest field of view possible to ensure you can see the entire length of the aneurysm. This will also allow you to determine which other arteries may be compromised by the aneurysm.

FIGURE 5.16.   Evaluating the involvement of significant landmarks. In this picture, the aneurysm is located at the level of the renal arteries, although the aneurysmal dilatation does not involve these arteries.

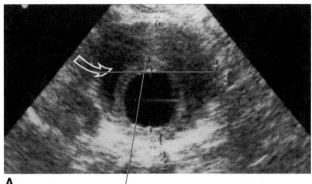

A

Abdominal aortic aneurysm with significant
thrombus like material in the lumen

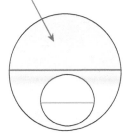

B

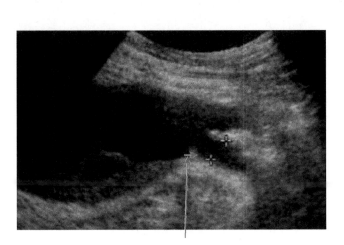

FIGURE 5.17.   Measuring the distance to the common iliac arteries and the diameter of these arteries. In this picture, the aneurysm (arrow) does not significantly involve the common iliac arteries, yet the aorta is clearly dilated up to the level of the bifurcation.

FIGURE 5.18.   Aneurysm with thrombus or plaque, special considerations. With this presentation, it is important to note the presence of the thrombus (or plaque) and to measure the diameter of the aneurysm (red line) and also that of the remaining lumen (green line).

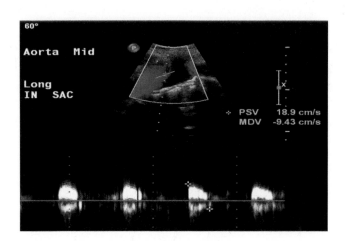

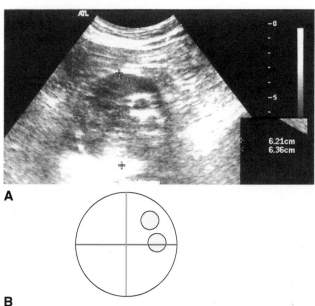

A

B

FIGURE 5.19. Evaluating flow in the aneurysm by Doppler. Distension of the lumen by an aneurysm may induce low flow and turbulence, which in turn may increase the risk for thrombosis.

FIGURE 5.20. This picture shows an aneurysm sac with an endograft.

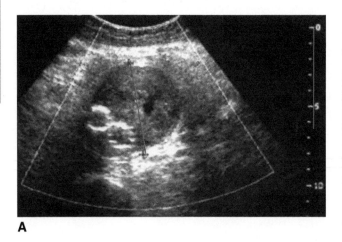

A

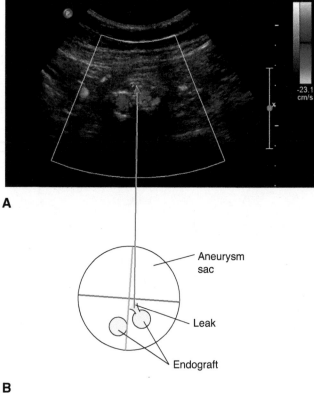

A

B

B

FIGURE 5.21. Infrarenal aortic aneurysm after endovascular repair (anterior approach, transverse view). The aneurysmal sac measures approximately 6 cm anteroposteriorly. The endograft shows the bifurcated portion deep inside the aneurysmal sac.

FIGURE 5.22. Small endoleak. The original aneurysmal sac is barely visible because of the organization of the thrombus which has now acquired an echogenicity similar to surrounding tissue. Power Doppler or lower color Doppler settings could be used to ensure that very small leaks (with low flow do not remain undetected).

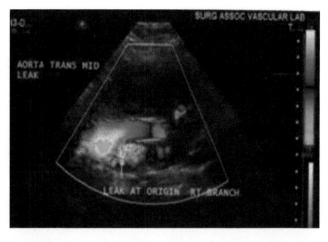

FIGURE 5.23.   Endoleak detected at the iliac "leg" connection of this composite endograft.

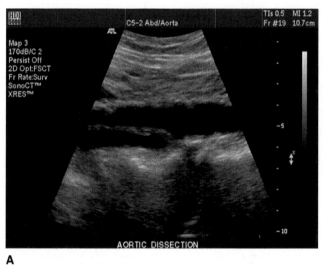

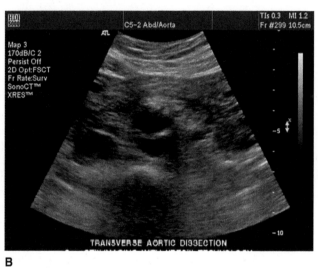

A

B

FIGURE 5.24.   Grayscale images in longitudinal and transverse views.

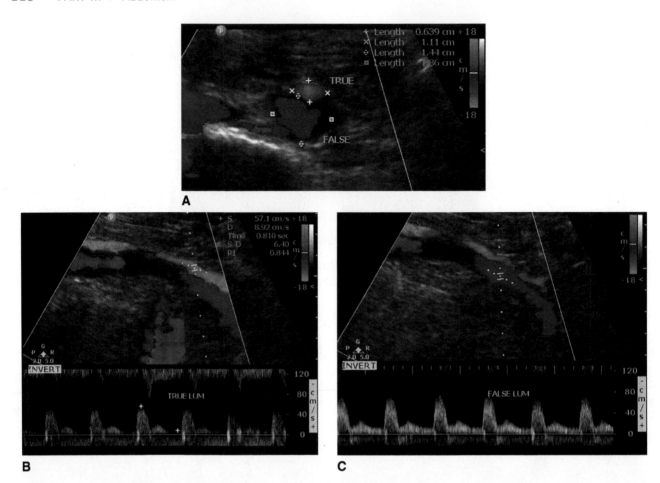

FIGURE 5.25.   Dissection of the abdominal aorta. A dissection usually occurs between the intima and media layers of an artery, creating two lumen where the flow can go. Figure A (in longitudinal view) and Figure B (in transverse view) are B mode pictures showing a thin line within the lumen of the vessels, the dissected portion. It is important to use every means possible to evaluate the extent of a dissection when present, particularly to evaluate if the dissection involves major branches of the aorta such as the renal arteries. A dissection can create a "flap" which may block flow to an artery and therefore an organ.

CHAPTER 5

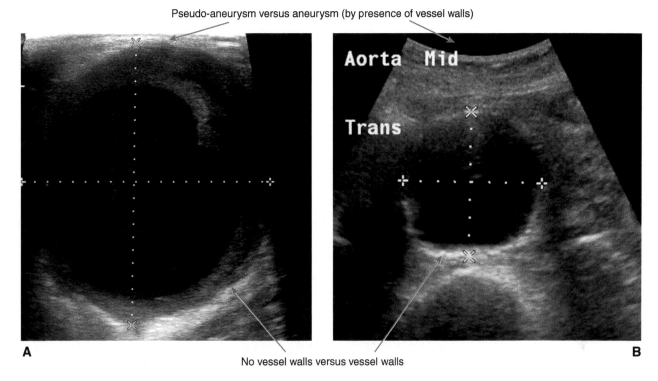

Pseudo-aneurysm versus aneurysm (by presence of vessel walls)

No vessel walls versus vessel walls

FIGURE 5.26. Comparing pseudoaneurysm to aneurysm by presence of vessel walls. A pseudoaneurysm is a false dilatation created by flow escaping from an artery and contained within the surrounding tissue. A pseudoaneurysm should not show sign of arterial layers.

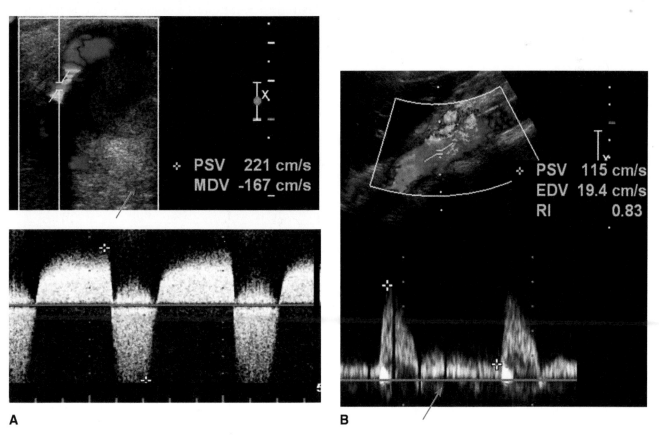

FIGURE 5.27. Comparing pseudoaneurysm to aneurysm by characteristics of Doppler waveforms. (A) Typical to-and-fro flow at the neck of the pseudoaneurysm versus (B) typical medium- to high-resistance arterial flow pattern in the aneurysm lumen.

Concluding Tips

Duplex ultrasound is a feasible technique to evaluate the aorta. This chapter focused on the evaluation of the aorta for the assessment of fusiform aneurysms. The rationales for this choice are explained in the earlier Tips/Rationale section. In this summative section, it is important to add that this choice is also supported by the rare occurrence of saccular aneurysms, particularly at the level of the infrarenal abdominal aorta. When present, they typically occur in the suprarenal portion of the abdominal aorta. They are often secondary to infection (from syphilis) or trauma (from nonpuncture blow to the abdomen). The last comment on saccular aneurysms will be a cautionary note. Due to their appearance (i.e., focal out-pouching of one portion of the aortic wall), they may be mistaken for pseudoaneurysms. The presence of a clearly defined wall and no neck and the patient's history should allow for proper identification.

Although duplex ultrasound has found its place in the screening and detection of aneurysms, its role in the evaluation of repair, particularly from endovascular techniques, remains to be clearly validated. The main drawbacks of endovascular grafts are endoleaks and endotension; however, both are difficult to evaluate by ultrasound. Although the results of endoleaks or endotension are somewhat easy to note, because they both will trigger an expansion of the aneurysm sac, the source may be difficult to visualize. The development and improvement of three-dimensional techniques and image reconstruction will likely make the use of duplex ultrasound more predominant for this purpose.

PART THREE: ABDOMEN

Testing the Mesenteric Circulation

Chapter Outline

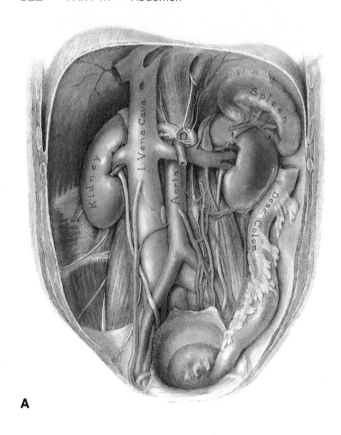

A

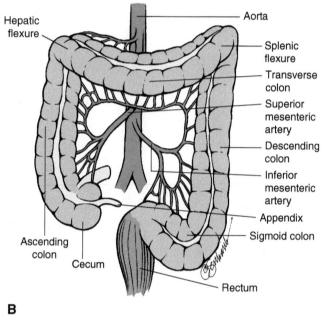

B

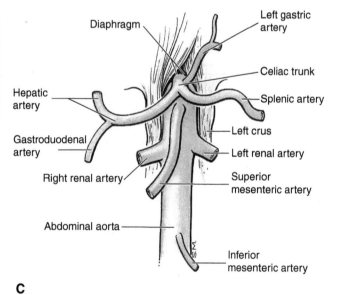

C

FIGURE 6.1.   (A) Relative position of the major organs in the abdomen and their vasculature (with the exclusion of the intestines). (B) Superior mesenteric artery (SMA) and inferior mesenteric artery (IMA) circulation. (C) Close up of the take-off position of the major branches of the abdominal aorta.

General Concepts in Mesenteric Circulation Evaluation

The splanchnic circulation includes all vessels leading to or draining the "inner" (which is the meaning of the word *splanchnic*) organs, which include the liver, the spleen, the stomach, the pancreas, all parts of the small intestine, and the colon.

This chapter will focus on part of the splanchnic circulation referred to as the mesenteric circulation, which is involved in the digestive system composed of all parts of the small intestine and colon. Therefore, this chapter will solely discuss the role of ultrasound in the investigation of abdominal pain suspicious for mesenteric ischemia. The hepatoportal circulation will be the subject of a subsequent chapter in this section of the book related to the abdominal vasculature.

It is also important to note here that this chapter will focus on the use of ultrasound for the diagnosis or exclusion of chronic mesenteric ischemia as the cause of abdominal pain. Indeed, due to the potentially fatal nature of acute mesenteric ischemia, ultrasound and, more specifically, duplex ultrasound are not deemed to be practical for such purpose.

Finally, although it is important to consider the roles of pathologies of arteries and veins in evaluating ischemia of the mesenteric system, it is important to note that thrombosis of mesenteric veins is relatively uncommon (and linked to other conditions such as malignancies and/or sepsis) and will often lead to acute ischemia.

Tips/Rationale

- Because of the complexity and anatomic variability of the splanchnic circulation, it is crucial to have a clear understanding of the anatomy and the roles of each of the major arteries and veins that will be under investigation in an examination for chronic mesenteric ischemia.
- The major arteries supplying the intestinal organs are the superior mesenteric artery (SMA) and inferior mesenteric artery (IMA), both ventral branches of the aorta.
- The SMA supplies the small intestine (including part of the duodenum, the jejunum, and ileum), ascending colon, and most of the transverse colon.
- The IMA supplies the remainder of the colon and terminates as paired hemorrhoidal arteries.
- Both the SMA and the IMA lead to a very rich supply of blood vessels somewhat encapsulating the intestinal organs and can thus form many anastomoses or provide collateral routes.
- The venous drainage is done through the superior mesenteric vein (SMV) and inferior mesenteric vein (IMV), which will form the portal venous system leading to the liver.
- The SMV follows a similar route as the SMA and will join the splenic vein to form the main portal vein.
- The IMV drains into the splenic vein before it joins the SMV to form the main portal vein.

- The celiac trunk (also known as celiac axis or celiac artery) branches into the common hepatic artery, the left gastric artery, and the splenic artery.

- The common hepatic artery branches out into the gastroduodenal and proper hepatic arteries, with the gastroduodenal artery leading to multiple branches supplying part of the stomach and the duodenum and jejunum and the proper hepatic artery supplying the liver.

- Because the gastroduodenal artery and its multiple branches may serve as important collateral routes for the supply of the intestinal tract, the investigation of the celiac trunk is an integral part of protocols for mesenteric ischemia.

- Because of this rich blood supply, arterial pathologies that would lead to chronic ischemia of the intestine and colon necessitate a drastic change of blood supply.

- It has been shown that ≥ 70% stenosis or occlusion of *at least two* of the major vessels (celiac, SMA, or IMA) or, in rarer cases, thrombosis of some of the corresponding veins (IMV, SMV) is necessary to lead to significant and symptomatic chronic mesenteric ischemia.

- Thus, the protocol for investigation (from the Intersocietal Commission for the Accreditation of Vascular Laboratory [ICAVL] standards) of chronic mesenteric ischemia is mainly limited to the celiac trunk, SMA, IMA, and adjacent aorta. When necessary and/or appropriate, for example in case of unusual anatomic distribution of branches (particularly of the hepatic arteries) or because of potential for collateral routes, the splenic and hepatic arteries may be included.

- Duplex ultrasound will be used to determine the vascular cause of chronic mesenteric ischemia, as well as to follow the success of treatment.

- Treatment of arterial etiology of chronic mesenteric ischemia is done via stenting of the stenosis when amenable, via endarterectomy (or removal of plaque), or, most often, via bypass graft from the aorta to a nondiseased portion of the SMA or IMA.

- Finally, the request for evaluating the mesenteric system may be based on nonspecific or intermittent pain not specifically pointing to a vascular etiology. As with all the tests described so far, a thorough patient history can point to the results. Without significant weight loss and specific and documented postprandial pain, it is very unlikely that a vascular etiology is the cause of the abdominal pain.

Protocol Algorithms

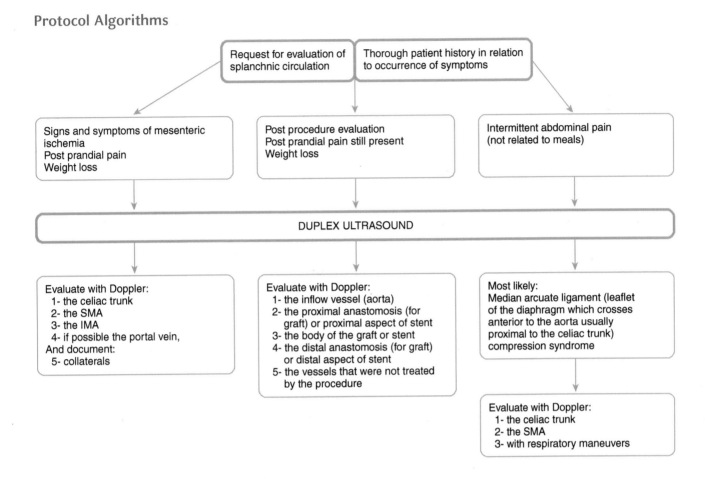

FIGURE 6.2.   Algorithm for examination of the mesenteric circulation.

Imaging Studies by Duplex

Test Preparation

- It is recommended that the patient fasts (as with most examinations involving the abdominal vasculature) for the baseline exam.

- It should be noted that most patients with chronic mesenteric ischemia will have experienced a significant weight loss from "fear" of eating due to postprandial pain and will present to the vascular laboratory fasting.

- Some laboratories include a preprandial (for baseline data) AND a postprandial examination. The postprandial examination is usually performed after the administration of a high-calorie drink to induce a heightened requirement for flow from digestion.

- The rationale is similar to that of exercising a patient on a treadmill to demonstrate the presence and/or the significance of claudication. Inducing the digestive process through a high-calorie drink will increase the blood flow in the celiac and SMA initially and may allow for a clearer demonstration of stenosis.

- However, a search on the internet about the practicality and usefulness of this digestion challenge has not yielded any recent publications (most publications on the topic are from the late 1980s through the mid-1990s), and the ICAVL does not mention such practice in its examination standards.

- One of the reasons for abandoning such practice is that patients presenting with true chronic mesenteric ischemia will describe progressive weight loss and fear of eating, already pointing to suboptimal calorie intake.

- In addition and most importantly, because chronic mesenteric ischemia requires, as explained earlier, that at least two of the three major arteries be significantly stenosed or occluded, the baseline (preprandial) exam will already demonstrate stenosis or occlusion when present, particularly with the technology advances in imaging and Doppler.

- Finally (and as a side note to consider in our role in health care), some have mentioned that inducing pain (because in true mesenteric ischemia, the high-calorie drink will surely trigger abdominal pain) is unwarranted because it does not add more information for diagnosis.

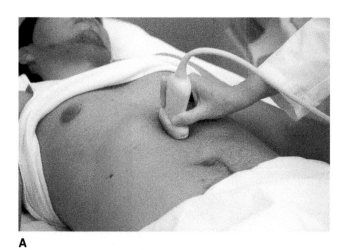

A

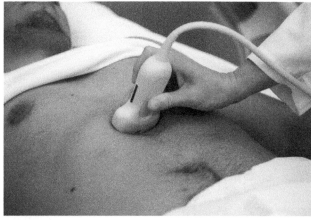

B

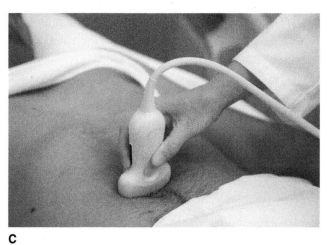

C

FIGURE 6.3.   There are not many options to view the vessels of the mesenteric system except to insonate the body from an anterior approach. The transducer will be moved distally to the iliac bifurcation (A,B) and back a few centimeters to identify the IMA (C).

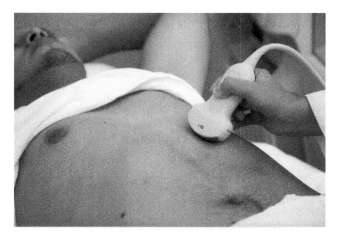

FIGURE 6.4.   To obtain a long axis image of the vessel, placing the transducer slightly lateral may improve the view. Gentle massage with the transducer may help in shifting intestinal gas and reduce acoustic shadowing.

Testing Sequence

The testing sequence should include:

- The identification of the celiac trunk, SMA, and IMA in transverse and longitudinal views.
- The identification of the aorta in transverse and longitudinal views noting the presence or absence of aneurysm and/or stenosis or occlusion.
- Doppler of the abdominal aorta at the level of the celiac/SMA and at the level of the IMA, in longitudinal view.
- The identification of the celiac trunk, SMA, and IMA in longitudinal view for documentation of flow with Doppler (although the origin itself of each of these vessels can often be better sampled by Doppler in a transverse view). The angle of insonation should remain as much as possible below 60°, and an angle of 0° may be used at the origin in a transverse view for some vessels such as the celiac trunk.
- The identification and documentation of flow with Doppler of the splenic and hepatic artery when appropriate, as described earlier.
- The identification and documentation of flow with Doppler of some of the veins, paying special attention to the direction of flow in addition to pattern of flow when appropriate, as described earlier.
- Additional documentation will pertain to evaluation when stenosis and/or occlusion of the main vessels are present and could be as follows:
  - Identification and/or note of collaterals
  - Doppler samples before and after stenosis (if feasible)
  - Other unusual findings (such as, but not limited to, aneurysms of branches and enlarged lymph nodes along the aorta)

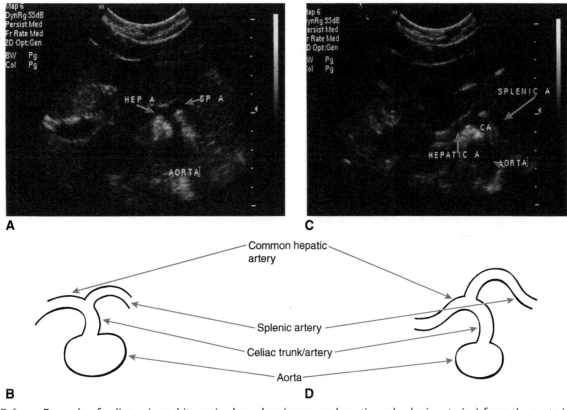

FIGURE 6.5. Example of celiac axis and its major branches (common hepatic and splenic arteries) from the aorta in a transverse view. Note: The left gastric artery, the third major branch of the celiac axis, is often not visualized by ultrasound.

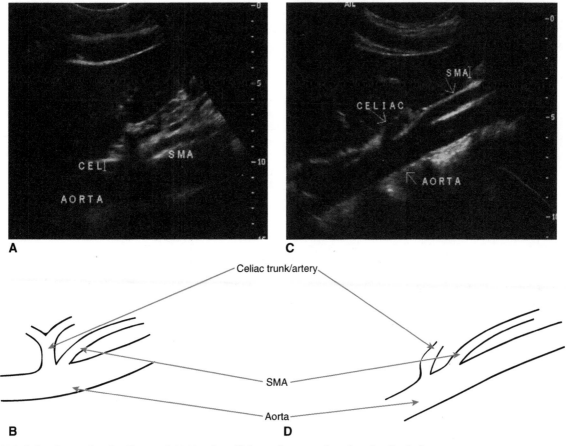

FIGURE 6.6. Example of celiac and SMA take-off from the aorta in a longitudinal view.

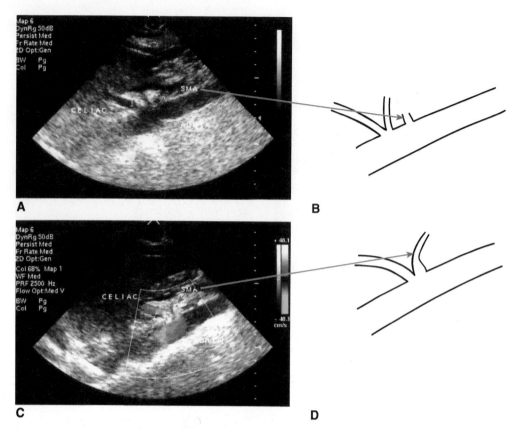

FIGURE 6.7.   Example of celiac and SMA take-off from the aorta in a longitudinal view.

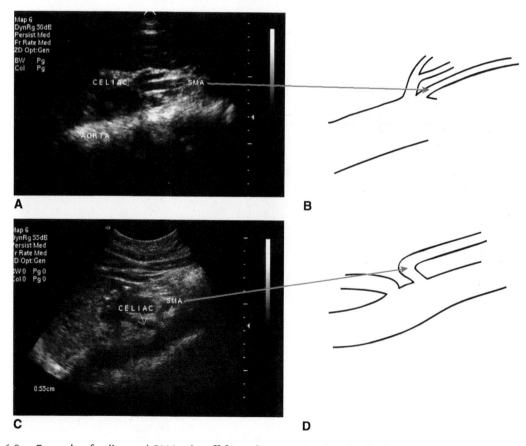

FIGURE 6.8.   Example of celiac and SMA take-off from the aorta in a longitudinal view.

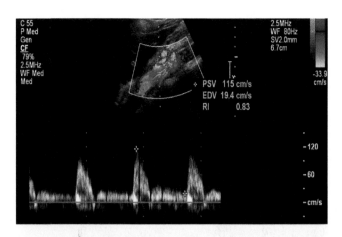

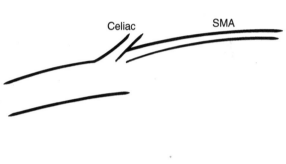

FIGURE 6.9. Normal velocities and Doppler waveforms in the aorta at the level of the SMA. The peak systolic velocity could be used to calculate a systolic celiac-to-aorta, SMA-to-aorta, and IMA-to-aorta ratio. However, note that there are no clearly established criteria using these ratios for the diagnosis of stenosis in the arteries of the mesenteric system. However, it is conceivable to study the possibility of using these ratios in a similar fashion for renal artery stenosis. Correlation analysis would be needed to ensure validity and accuracy before use.

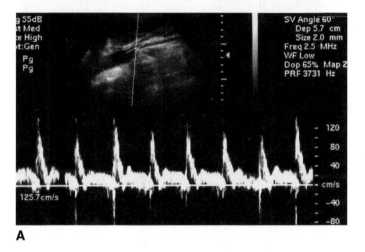

A

B

FIGURE 6.10. Normal Doppler waveforms and velocities at the celiac trunk origin. Celiac trunk/artery preprandial. The peak systolic velocity is recorded at 125 cm/s. The late diastolic velocity is < 40 cm/s with slight flow reversal in early diastole, which points to medium to high resistance for this vessel (somewhat comparable to an external carotid artery [ECA]).

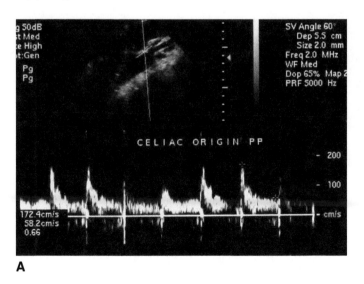

A

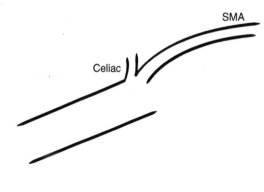

B

FIGURE 6.11. Normal Doppler waveforms and velocities at the SMA preprandial. Celiac trunk/artery postprandial. The peak systolic velocity is recorded at 172 cm/s. The late diastolic velocity is now 58 cm/s, and the slight reversal of flow in early diastole is not visible anymore. This points to a slight change to lower resistance postprandial (closer to a common carotid artery [CCA] or internal carotid artery [ICA]).

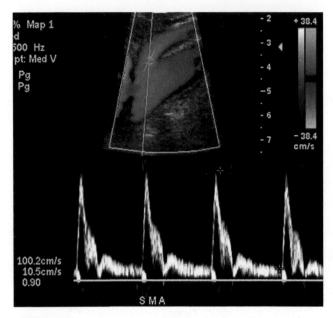

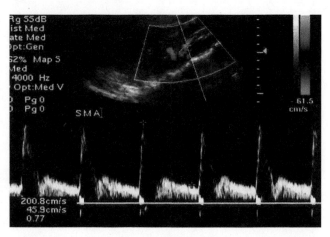

FIGURE 6.12.   Normal Doppler waveforms and velocities at the SMA preprandial (before a meal). The peak systolic velocity is recorded at 100 cm/s, and the end diastolic velocity is 10 cm/s. The waveforms are typical of high-resistance flow, and the resistive index is 0.90 (comparable to an ECA waveform).

FIGURE 6.13.   Normal Doppler waveforms and velocities at the IMA postprandial (after a meal). SMA Doppler postprandial. The peak systolic velocity is recorded at 200 cm/s, and the end diastolic velocity is 46 cm/s, with a much lower resistive index than observed preprandial. The waveforms are typical of lower resistance with higher flow in diastole.

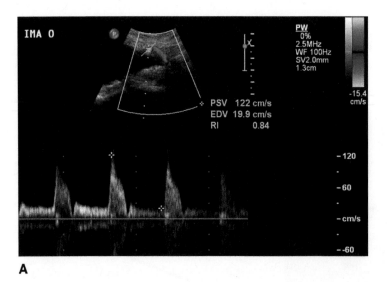

A

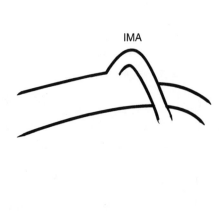

B

FIGURE 6.14.   Take off of the IMA from the ventral aspect of the aorta. Doppler waveforms and flow pattern preprandial or early postprandial are shown. Note: The IMA can be difficult to visualize. It usually has a smaller diameter than the celiac or SMA. The best approach is to scan the aorta to the iliac bifurcation, then slowly scan more proximally from the iliac bifurcation with color Doppler and look for a ventral or slightly anterolateral branch (to the left); therefore, a slightly right lateral approach is best suited, and the IMA would appear superior to the aorta, as in this image.

Results and Interpretation

TABLE 6.1: Flow Pattern and Velocity Criteria: Comparison of Normal and Abnormal Findings by Vessel

	Celiac Trunk	SMA	IMA
Normal Finding			
Flow pattern	Low-resistance pattern pre- and postprandial with very minimal variations	High-resistance pattern preprandial changing to low-resistance pattern postprandial	Same as SMA, although the low-resistance pattern will be seen later during the digestion process (since the IMA supplies the colon)
Velocities	Between 100 and 150 cm/s; rule is < 200 cm/s	< 250 cm/s (with only slight variations in peak systole between pre- and postprandial states); the diastolic flow velocity will increase significantly postprandial	Same as SMA
> 60% Stenosis			
Flow pattern	Continued low-resistance pattern pre- and postprandial with minimal variations	Same characteristics as in normal state, although severe stenosis may induce distal vasodilation, which may translate into a slight increase in diastolic velocities because of the slight decrease in distal resistance preprandial	Same as SMA
Velocities	> 220 cm/s	> 275 cm/s	Same as SMA
Occlusion			
Flow pattern	Look for increased flow in the SMA and IMA, as well as anatomic variants and collaterals	Look for increased flow in celiac and IMA, as well as anatomic variants and collaterals	Look for increased flow in celiac and SMA, as well as collaterals

CHAPTER 6

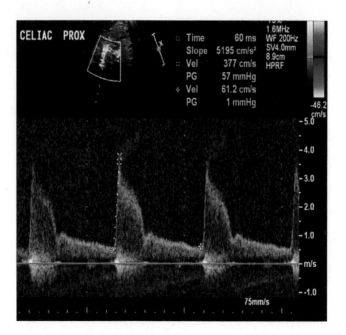

FIGURE 6.15. Severe stenosis (> 60%) at the level of the proximal celiac trunk (axis, artery). The peak systolic velocities are recorded at > 300 cm/s.

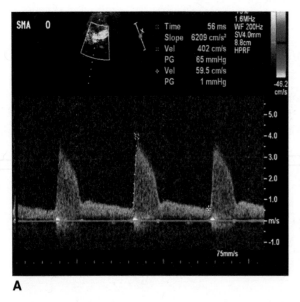

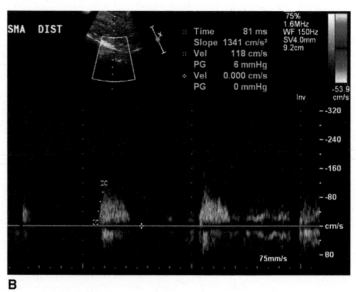

A   B

FIGURE 6.16. Severe stenosis (> 60%) at the origin of the SMA. The peak systolic velocities were recorded > 400 cm/s. The image is followed by evaluation of a more distal segment of the SMA, distal to the stenosis, where significant decreases in peak systolic velocities are noted. The waveforms display a high-resistance pattern suggesting an exam preprandial. As noted in the text, we can appreciate here the reliability of demonstrating significant disease without having to resort to a caloric challenge.

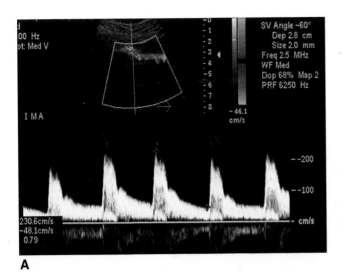
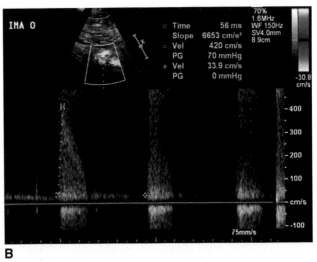

A   **B**

FIGURE 6.17.   Greater than 60% stenosis at the origin of the IMA. Note the turbulence at the origin of the vessel seen by color Doppler and the increase of peak systolic velocities to > 220 cm/s (recorded at 230 cm/s) in the first picture and to > 400 cm/s in the second picture. The diastolic flow velocity, on the other hand, did not significantly change from the velocities observed in the absence of disease in the first picture but is low in the second picture, which may imply that the exam was done preprandial.

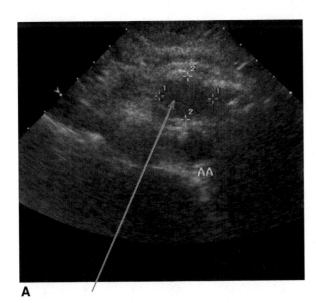
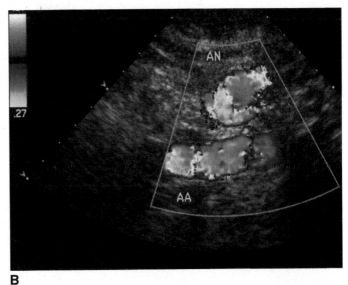

A   **B**

FIGURE 6.18.   Unusual aneurysm at the pancreaticoduodenal artery. (A) A large round structure is noted superior to the aorta in this transverse picture taken at the level of the SMA. (B) The longitudinal view at the same level shows again a dilated/aneurysmal vessel superior (anterior) to the aorta. The diagnosis in this case was not made until an angiogram was performed. The aneurysmal artery was found to be the pancreaticoduodenal artery, which served as a collateral route to supply flow to the splenic and common hepatic arteries as well as to reconstitute the SMA, due to occlusion at the origin of the celiac trunk and SMA.

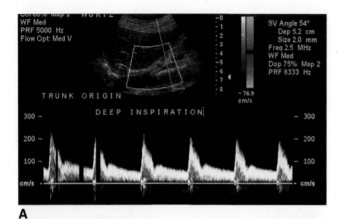

A

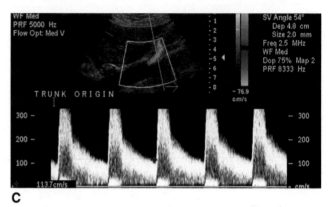

B

FIGURE 6.19.   Compression of the celiac trunk origin by the median arcuate ligament, which is also known as median arcuate syndrome. During inspiration (inhaling phase of respiration), the celiac trunk exhibits normal flow velocities (top picture) with < 200 cm/s in peak systole. During deep expiration (exhaling phase of respiration), the median arcuate ligament leaflets are shifted downward, creating a temporary compression of the origin of the celiac trunk and mimicking a stenosis (two bottom pictures). The peak systolic velocity is now recorded at > 300 cm/s. Note: It may be necessary to have the patient in a sitting or standing position and performing deep expiration to demonstrate this syndrome. There seems to be a slight prevalence in women.

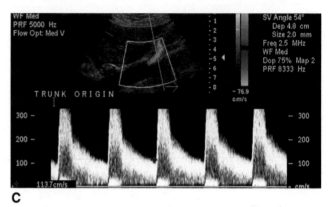

C

FIGURE 6.20.   Splenic artery and veins. The main word of caution here is that the spleen and its vasculature can easily display a similar pattern as the left kidney.

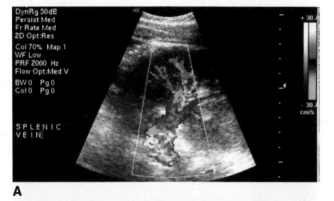

A

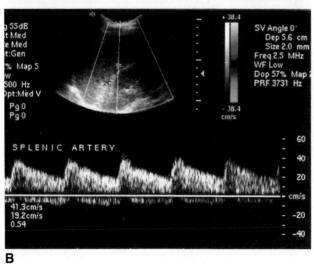

B

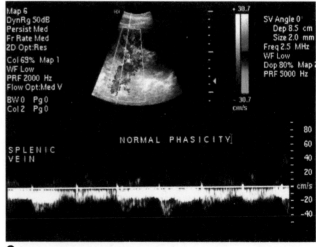

C

CHAPTER 6

Concluding Tips

Abdominal pain or pain suffered or perceived in the abdominal region can have many etiologies and be linked to many pathologies. The intestine and colon are richly supplied organs by three major arteries and a great expanse of collateral routes. Therefore, mesenteric ischemia is not as common of a consequence of arterial stenosis as ischemia in other organs of the body, even though atherosclerosis and subsequent stenosis of the origin of the celiac or SMA are not uncommon in patients prone to atherosclerotic disease.

In addition, the small intestine and colon are able to tolerate decreased flow for a long period of time. The main reason for this special ability is that under normal circumstances, only approximately one-fifth of the capillaries are open at one time; that is, the mesenteric system is able to perform its metabolic function perfectly well at one-fifth of its full capacity!

A thorough patient history, particularly in regard to the occurrence of pain and documentation of weight loss, will be the most reliable clue suggesting chronic mesenteric ischemia. Remember that patients with acute mesenteric ischemia should really not present in the vascular laboratory due to the life-threatening nature of the condition. When the examination is requested for nonspecific pain, ultrasound may not be (or should not be) the best screening method. However, ultrasound is helpful in the documentation median arcuate compression syndrome.

PART THREE: ABDOMEN

Testing the Renal Circulation

Chapter Outline

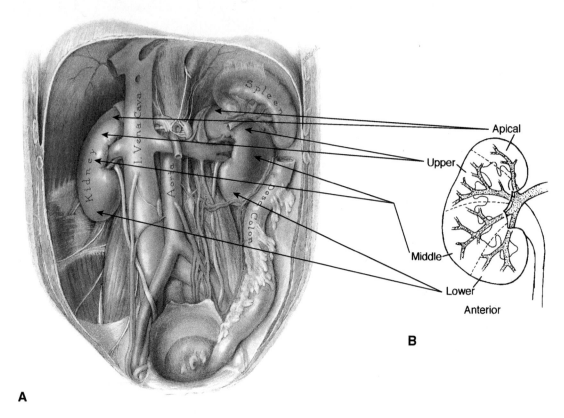

FIGURE 7.1.   Internal anatomic position of the kidneys in the retroperitoneal space. Kidney cross section correlates to the in vivo areas of interest during ultrasound examination.

General Concepts in Renal Circulation Evaluation

Although duplex ultrasound has become, in many laboratories, a routine examination for the vasculature of the kidneys, there are still debates regarding its accuracy. Indeed, in comparison to other widely accepted imaging modalities such as angiogram, magnetic resonance angiogram (MRA), or computed tomography angiogram (CTA), duplex ultrasound has some limitations, particularly with the evaluation of some anatomic variants such as double arterial system or other accessory arteries. Therefore, it is felt that even when disease is not present in the main (and sometimes only visible) renal artery, ultrasound does not have the capability to totally exclude disease in nonvisualized accessory or double renal arteries. The goal of this manual is not to enter into these debates, but these questions should remind us that the purpose of diagnostic imaging is to offer information not readily available by physical exams for planning the best course of action for the patient. As such we should always remember, accept, and admit the potential limitations of some tests.

With that said, technologic advances and indirect measurements have allowed for duplex ultrasound to offer a safe testing modality for patients with suspected renal insufficiency and/or hypertension, as well as for follow-up of treatments by angioplasty and stenting, or even transplantation.

Tips/Rationale

The following tips do not follow a particular order of importance.

- Although these bilateral organs are rather easily identified by ultrasound (they really do have a kidney shape!), locating them may still be challenging.
  - The liver on the right but also, to some extent, the spleen on the left can be used as an acoustic window.
  - Remember that these organs are retroperitoneal, so using an anterior or ventral scanning approach is probably not the most efficient.
  - Finally, keep in mind that the kidneys are relatively high in the abdomen and not nicely positioned on a vertical axis. The right and left kidneys are in the mid portion of the right and left upper quadrants or lower portion of the right and left hypochondriac to upper portion of the right and left lumbar regions, respectively. The upper poles of both kidneys are at the level of the celiac trunk or T12-T13 on each side of the vertebral column. The left kidney is usually slightly superior compared with the right kidney. Both kidneys have an oblique position, with the upper poles slightly more posterior than the lower poles.
- Once the kidneys are located and identified, the next challenge rests in the examination of the vasculature, including both the veins and arteries. Here again, a clear vision of the anatomic position of the main vessels and possible variants will allow for "creative" and tailored scanning approaches.
  - Due to the relative position of the great vessels (i.e., inferior vena cava [IVC] and aorta), the right renal artery is normally posterior to the IVC, whereas the left renal vein courses anterior to the aorta.
  - Both renal veins are mostly anterior to the arteries and drain in the IVC.
  - The presence of accessory renal arteries and double arteries and early bifurcation of the main renal arteries proximal to the renal hilum are not uncommon.
  - In addition, due to the complex embryologic development of the venous system with the IVC, unusual configuration and position of the renal veins can exist (particularly on the left), such as retroaortic left renal vein or aortic collar (where two veins or two branches encircle the aorta before draining in the IVC).
  - Finally, although rare, some congenital anomalies may lead to unusual vasculature. For example, with horseshoe kidneys (kidneys fused at the lower pole), it is not unusual to have multiple main renal arteries and veins. In case of ectopic pelvic kidneys, the renal artery and vein will be located much more distal as a branch of the aorta for the former and tributary of the IVC for the latter (sometimes at the level of the iliac bifurcation).

- Duplex ultrasound is a perfectly well-suited technology for the follow-up of kidney transplants. In these cases, the kidney is usually positioned rather superficially in the right pelvic fossa, and the donor artery and vein are anastomosed with the recipient right common or external iliac artery and vein in an end-to-side fashion. Make sure to have the proper history, and do not confuse a transplant for an ectopic kidney.

■ A few important and additional tips are as follows:

- Kidneys come in pairs, so always examine both. However, people can easily live with one kidney, and as seen before in very rare instances, one kidney may be in an unusual location, so if you have doubt, question the person who should know best—the patient.

- Make sure to inform the patient that the exam may be long and may require him or her to change position as best as he or she can.

- Be patient, thorough, and vigilant throughout the exam.

Protocol Algorithms

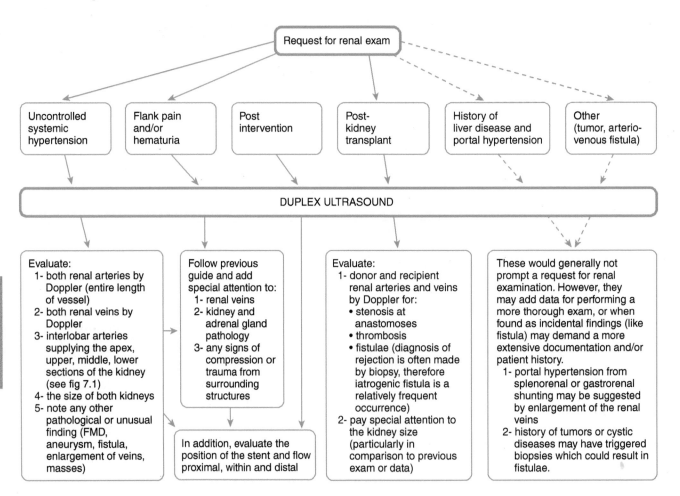

FIGURE 7.2.   Algorithm with recommendations for examination of the renal vasculature.

CHAPTER 7

Imaging Studies by Duplex

Test Preparation

As with any test, the idea is to find the most adequate position for performing the exam and for the patient's comfort (although the sonographer's comfort should not be compromised either). Positions that would allow for the greatest opening of the rib cage and not disrupt the breathing rhythm should be considered and/or chosen, particularly in challenging exams.

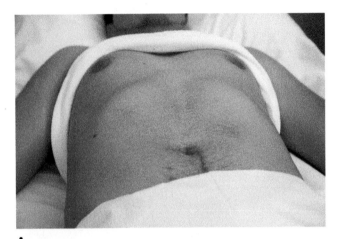

A

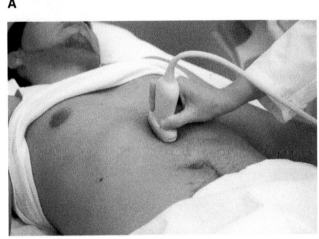

B

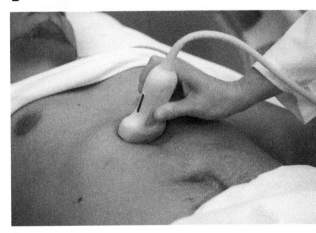

C

FIGURE 7.3.   Patient in supine position. This view is almost necessary independent of the possible challenges to examine the aorta and the origin of both renal arteries by Doppler.

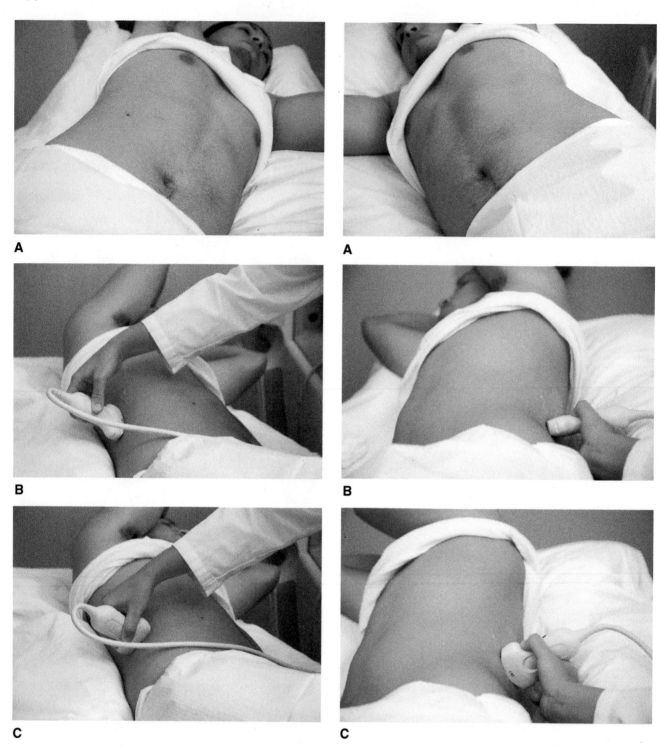

A

B

C

A

B

C

FIGURE 7.4. Patient in left lateral decubitus position. This position allows for maximizing the view of the right kidney, both in longitudinal and transverse, using the liver as an acoustic window.

FIGURE 7.5. Patient in right lateral decubitus position. This position allows one to obtain views of the left kidney by using the spleen as an acoustic window.

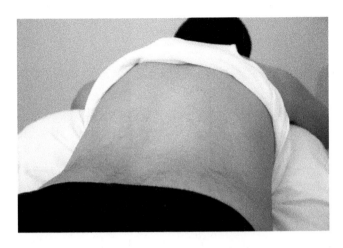

FIGURE 7.6.   Patient in prone position. This may be the optimal position to examine the left kidney. However, it is important to keep in mind that most patients will not be able to maintain such a position (mostly because of difficulty breathing).

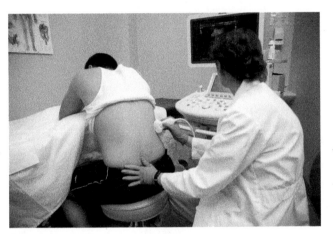

A

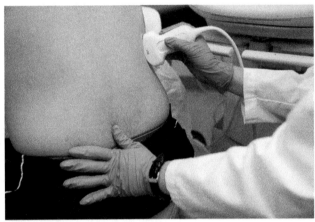

B

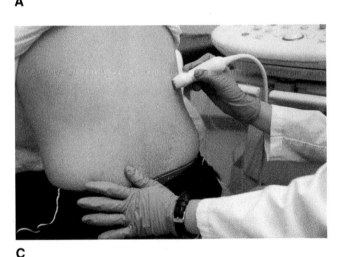

C

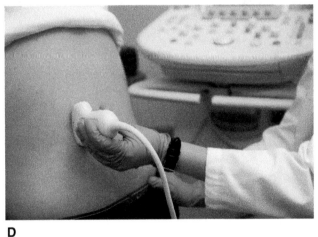

D

FIGURE 7.7.   The position depicted here (patient sitting with arm resting on the examination table) is rarely used (one lab in Fort Myers, Florida, where my colleague and associate professor at NSU, Samuel Yoders, MHSc, RVT works, uses it and a lab in Tucson, Arizona uses a modified version). This technique is now widely used in our teaching protocol at Nova Southeastern University in Fort Lauderdale, Florida. This position offers many great advantages: 1) it decreases the movement of the kidneys with breathing, 2) it removes the acoustic problems encountered from the intestine from an anterior approach, and 3) it is very comfortable for both the patient and sonographer. One of the disadvantages is that on large patients it may not allow for viewing the origin of the renal arteries. It also requires a little bit of a learning curve from more standards and widely used positions. (Continued)

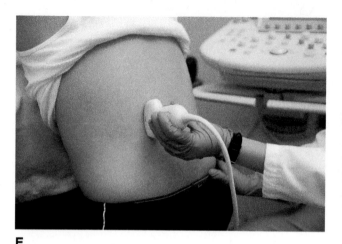

E

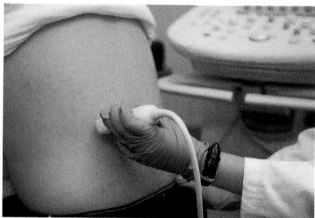

F

FIGURE 7.7.   (Continued)

Testing Sequence

The testing sequence should include, at a minimum, the following:

- The identification of the right and left kidneys in a longitudinal view of each kidney for measurements of the length of the organ from pole to pole (for this, remember that the kidneys are not positioned vertically in the body).

- The visualization of the aorta (the entire abdominal portion) to:
  - Exclude aneurismal and/or occlusive disease
  - Measure the peak systolic velocity at the level of the renal arteries (in a longitudinal view)

- The identification and visualization of both renal arteries (as well as accessory arteries) to obtain Doppler samples at the origin of the vessels, the mid portion of the vessel, and the distal portion of the vessel (at entrance to the hilum). Take a Doppler sample in the renal veins also. This portion of the exam is very likely to require moving the patient in different positions. Therefore, try to obtain whatever is possible in one position, and then move the patient. Basically avoid moving the patient back and forth (he or she may become frustrated and so will you!).

- Scan the parenchyma and note any pathologies (such as mass or cyst), and then turn color Doppler or power Doppler as well as your pulse Doppler to sweep through every pole and region (this will be part of your indirect measurements if you fail to clearly visualize the origin of the renal artery). This step is important if the patient has had a biopsy of the kidney tissue. Because of high-vascularization arteriovenous fistulae or pseudoaneurysms may result after a biopsy.

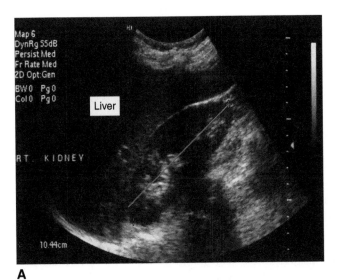
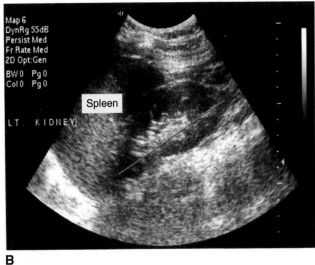

A   **B**

FIGURE 7.8.   Measuring the length, along its long axis, of the kidneys. Identify the right and left kidneys and position in a long axis to determine the length pole to pole. In an adult, the kidneys should measure at least 10 cm in length. There should not be significant difference between the right and left kidneys in term of size, although the left kidney may be 1/2 cm smaller than the right. Any kidneys measuring < 9 cm should heighten suspicion for significant vascular compromise, and any kidneys measuring > 13 cm should be suspicious for other pathologies. In a true long axis, the renal pelvis should be visible, meaning that there should be a visible break in the cortex at the mid pole.

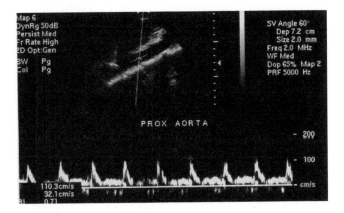

FIGURE 7.9.   Measuring the velocities of the proximal to mid aorta, in longitudinal view. After scanning the entire length of the abdominal aorta to ensure that aneurysmal or significant occlusive diseases are not present, flow velocities are obtained at or proximal to the level of the renal artery origins. The Doppler sample will be placed at mid stream and parallel to the vessel walls, and a Doppler angle of 60° or less should be used. The velocities in the aorta will be an integral part of the diagnostic criteria to determine the degree of stenosis if present. In addition, the Doppler waveform characteristics may point to more proximal pathologies, such as coarctation of the aorta, if the waveforms exhibit a significant delay in systole.

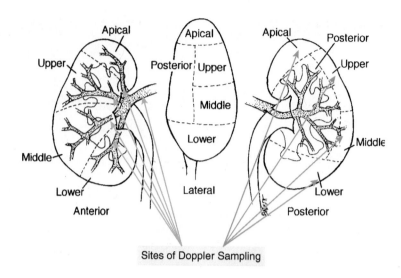

FIGURE 7.10.   This schematic representation of the kidneys demonstrates where the Doppler sample should be obtained.

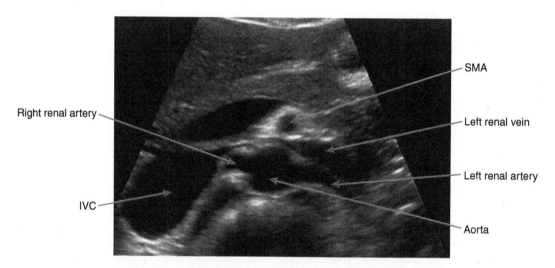

FIGURE 7.11.   This view allows you to obtain data for one-third of the exam. You can evaluate by Doppler the origin of both the right and left renal arteries, the left renal vein, and, by rotating your transducer in a longitudinal axis, the aorta (needed to calculate the renal-to-aorta ratio [RAR]). One of the best approaches to identify the position of the right and left renal artery is an anterior scanning approach in a transverse view. The SMA can serve as a landmark, and the renal arteries take off will usually be within 1.5 cm distally. This image represents a typical position of the right and left renal arteries in this approach, with the origin/take off of the right renal artery at approximately 10 o'clock and the left renal artery between 3 and 4 o'clock. This view would allow you to obtain Doppler sample at the origin of the right and left renal arteries and in the left renal vein.

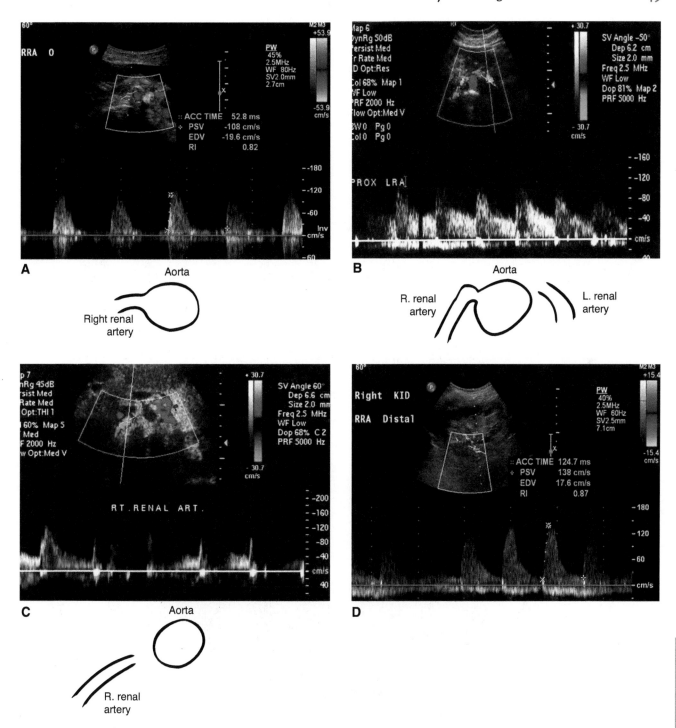

FIGURE 7.12. Obtaining a Doppler sample at different levels in the renal arteries. Doppler sampling should start at the origin of the renal artery. The artery should be followed toward the kidney to obtain velocities in the proximal, mid, and distal portions.

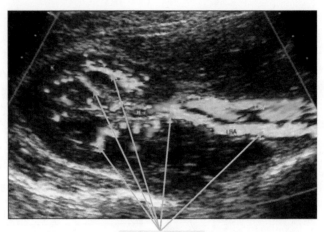

Doppler samples

FIGURE 7.13.   Alternate view to obtain Doppler sample in the renal artery and at the hilum. Transverse view of the mid portion of the kidney at the hilum. This view may allow you to follow back the renal arteries to their origin at the aorta if an anterior view did not permit you to do so. This view (transverse at the level of the renal hilum) offers a great opportunity to obtain Doppler samples in several key sites within one picture. The vasculature of the parenchyma is assessed here at the level of the mid pole of the kidney.

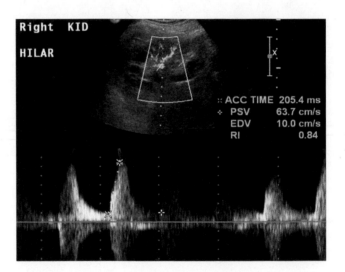

FIGURE 7.14.   In this picture the kidney is viewed along its long axis with the Doppler sample at the level of the renal pelvis. The Doppler sample should be moved to several sites (in a "fan shape" motion) to assess velocities in arteries going to all poles (upper, mid, and lower). This technique can also allow for identification of accessory or multiple renal arteries (indirectly). Indeed, like the branches of a tree, one main renal artery divides into smaller branches to feed all portions of the organ. With accessory arteries or multiple renal arteries, you may see different patterns where one pole will appear to be fed by an artery other than the main renal artery.

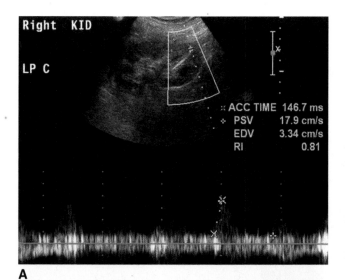

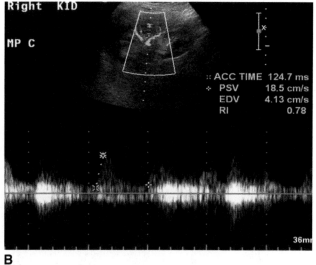

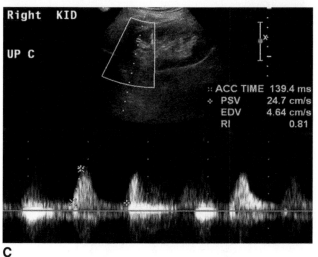

A

B

FIGURE 7.15.   Obtaining Doppler samples in the parenchyma of all poles. Doppler sampling should be done in representative arteries at the lower pole, mid pole, and upper pole of the kidneys. Although not represented here, power Doppler can sometimes greatly enhance areas to sample in the parenchyma. Note here how the sonographer has used the equipment's tools by reducing the sector width and focusing it only to the area being interrogated by Doppler. Courtesy of Samuel Yoders, MHSc, RVT.

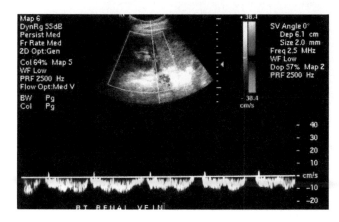

C

FIGURE 7.16.   Obtaining Doppler samples in the renal veins. A minimum of one Doppler sample in the right and left renal veins is necessary to exclude venous thrombosis but is also necessary for an indirect appreciation and understanding of other pathologies. Indeed, the left renal vein may become distended with increased flow in splenorenal or gastrorenal shunting in portal hypertension or after iatrogenic or otherwise arteriovenous fistula. The Doppler signal should show phasicity with respiration.

Results and Interpretation

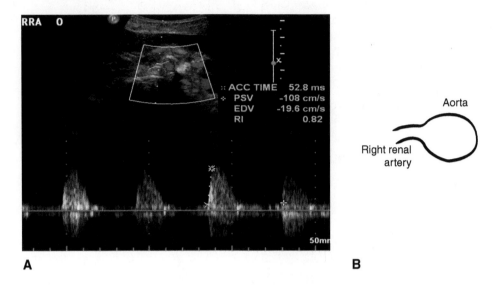

A   **B**

FIGURE 7.17. Interpreting Doppler waveforms and velocities. Interpretation: Peak systolic velocity (PSV) = 108 cm/s (between 70 and 130 cm/s or < 180 cm/s are accepted normal velocities in the main renal artery). Using a PSV of 100 cm/s in the aorta, the renal-to-aortic ratio (RAR) = 1.08. (RAR > 3.5 would indicate a > 60% stenosis assuming no disease was found in the aorta. Here the RAR is < 2.0 and the peak systolic velocities are < 180 cm/s which suggests no evidence of significant stenosis). The acceleration time here is 0.53 seconds or 53 milliseconds (rounded from 52.8 seen on the picture). The acceleration time should be under 0.7 seconds or 70 milliseconds. Courtesy of Samuel Yoders, MHSc, RVT.

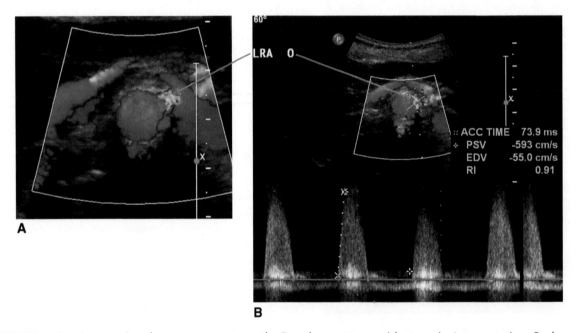

A

B

FIGURE 7.18. Interpreting the measurements on the Doppler spectrum with stenosis. Interpretation: Peak systolic velocity (PSV) = 593 cm/s (by the University of Washington criteria, PSVs > 180 cm/s are indicative of > 60% stenosis, with consideration of the renal-to-aortic ratio [RAR]). The PSV in the aorta was 150 cm/s, so the RAR = 3.9, also correlating with a > 60% (or hemodynamically significant) stenosis. Acceleration time (AT) = 0.74 s or 74 ms, which is within normal. The AT will take its full significance in the poststenotic segment to evaluate the impact on flow reduction and ultimately organ perfusion of the stenosis. Courtesy of Samuel Yoders, MHSc, RVT.

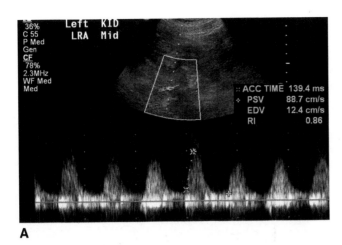
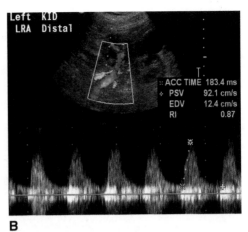

A **B**

FIGURE 7.19. Understanding the use of acceleration time (AT) and resistive index (RI) with stenosis. Interpretation: The velocities in the mid and distal left renal artery in these pictures are typical of the scenario observed distal to a stenosis. The ATs of 1.39 s or 139 ms in the mid renal artery and 1.83 s or 183 ms in the distal renal artery are representative of the delay to reach peak systole, due to decreased flow from the significant proximal stenosis. The RI (Peak Systolic Velocity – End Diastolic Velocity/Peak Systolic Velocity) of 0.86 and 0.87 is showing increased resistance, which may indicate deteriorating renal function (the RI should be < 0.70). Courtesy of Samuel Yoders, MHSc, RVT.

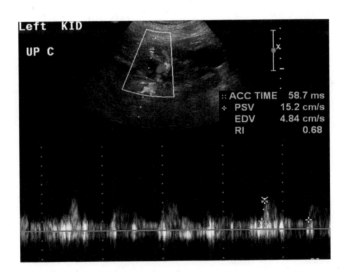

FIGURE 7.20. Using resistive index (RI) in the parenchyma as indirect measurement. Doppler sampling of the smaller arteries at the level of the parenchyma can offer indirect evaluation, particularly when the main renal artery is not well visualized. The RI (which should be < 0.70) can give an indication of the significance of a more proximal (and nonvisualized) stenosis on the overall perfusion and thus function of the kidney. However, this needs to be taken with great caution. In this example, the stenosis at the origin of the left renal artery is > 60%, yet the RI in the parenchyma does not reflect functional changes.

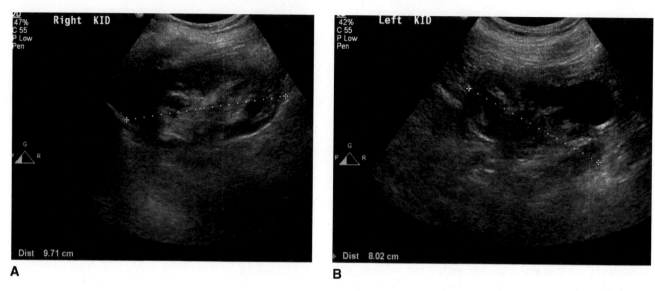

A　　　　　　　　　　　　　　　　　　　　　**B**

FIGURE 7.21. Using size discrepancy between kidneys as indirect measurement of stenosis. Kidney size or difference in kidney size is also an indirect method of evaluation of nonvisualized or poorly visualized stenosis or occlusion of the main renal artery. In this case, there is a > 1.5-cm difference in the length of the kidney (with the right within normal limits for an adult, but with the left significantly smaller and at a size suspicious for decreased function from decreased perfusion). Indeed, the left renal artery stenosis in this case has a > 60% stenosis at its origin.

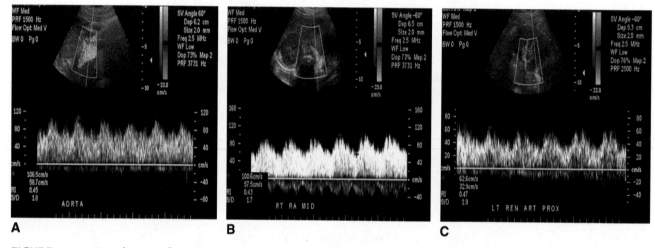

A　　　　　　　　　　　　**B**　　　　　　　　　　　　**C**

FIGURE 7.22. Doppler waveform characteristics in proximal aortic coarctation. The shape of the Doppler waveforms in a series and in multiple vessels should be worrisome. In all of these pictures, the resistive index (RI) is low at approximately 0.4. Although the suprarenal aorta and both renal arteries should display low resistance, the rounded waveforms and delay to peak systole suggest a more proximal problem. One possible diagnosis here is a coarctation of the descending aorta. This condition presents with a stricture of the aorta in the thorax, which reduces flow distally. Similar waveforms would be detected in the lower extremities with probably low ABI.

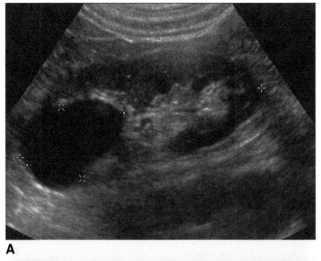

A

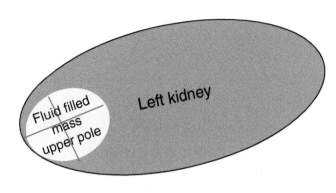

B

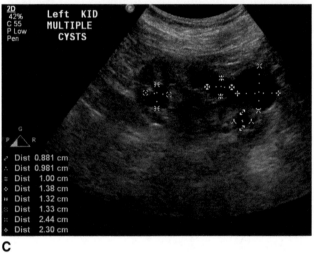

C

FIGURE 7.23. Fluid-filled mass in kidneys. Any incidental findings need to be reported. In addition, the arterial and venous Doppler signals in the vicinity of the mass should be assessed to rule out arteriovenous fistula, pseudoaneurysm, or hematoma.

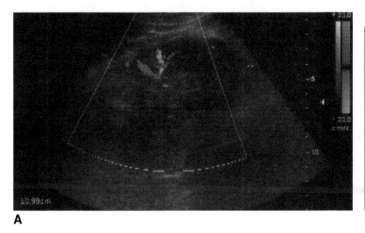

A

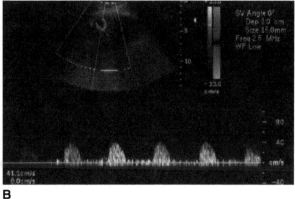

B

FIGURE 7.24. Ectopic kidney. This image represents an ectopic right kidney. The kidney was found in the pelvic region. Note how superficial the structure is and how there is no visible portion of the liver (compare to Fig. 7.8). Obtaining a detailed history from the patient and thinking "outside the box" were crucial for the sonographer to find this "wandering" kidney! Courtesy of Jeffrey Bradley, BHSc, RVT.

Concluding Tips

The examination of the renal vasculature is challenging. There is no doubt about it (unless you deal with a very young population, without intestines and great acoustic properties!). The best tip is to practice, first in a controlled setting in school on your classmates and then as much as possible in clinical settings. Nonetheless, even a seasoned sonographer will have to face challenges, so following are some additional tips:

- Find the best position (for you and for the patient) for imaging the particular patient you are dealing with.
- Do not be afraid to press rather hard, but warn the patient, particularly in your anterior/ventral approach.
- Be thorough and patient; however, recognize the limitations of the technique itself and also the patient (not everyone is "sonogenic").
- Keep in mind that you may not get those poster-perfect pictures, so take what you get when you get it; two waveforms in the spectrum that would allow you to understand what is happening are better than none.
- Remember that you can use some "indirect" measurements, such as the resistivity index (RI), the acceleration time, and a qualitative analysis of Doppler waveforms throughout the organ, to guide your interpretation.

PART THREE: ABDOMEN

Testing the Hepatoportal Circulation

Chapter Outline

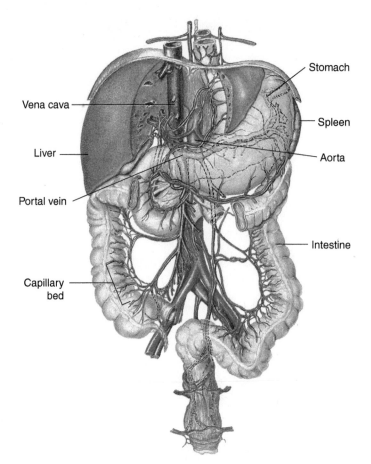

Vena cava

Liver

Portal vein

Capillary
bed

Stomach

Spleen

Aorta

Intestine

FIGURE 8.1.   Vessels and
organs of the upper abdomen
with hepatoportal circulation.

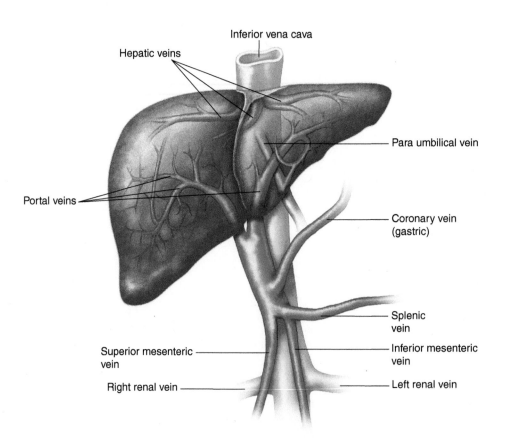

Inferior vena cava

Hepatic veins

Para umbilical vein

Portal veins

Coronary vein
(gastric)

Splenic
vein

Superior mesenteric
vein

Inferior mesenteric
vein

Right renal vein

Left renal vein

FIGURE 8.2.   Vessels of the
hepatoportal circulation.

General Concepts in Hepatoportal Circulation

This chapter (as well as the dialysis access chapter) differs slightly from the others in this book. It will lead to understanding the evaluation of a treatment option, known as TIPS or transjugular intrahepatic portosystemic shunt, used for some of the consequences of portal hypertension.

To understand the rationale for and the potential findings with TIPS, the chapter includes an overview of the anatomy and physiology of the vasculature of the liver and normal findings in the hepatoportal circulation.

Portal hypertension results from increased pressure in the portal venous system of the liver, preventing or impeding flow from this system (the splanchnic or digestive system) from entering the liver.

Portal hypertension can result from many different conditions affecting the liver or the vasculature of the liver (see Table 8.1), the main one being cirrhosis, and is characterized by portal venous pressure of at least 10 to 12 mm Hg (normal is < 5 mm Hg).

Independent of the etiology of portal hypertension, one of the most devastating complications is the development of varices mainly around the stomach or esophagus, which may lead to massive hemorrhage (due to the fragility of these veins from the limited ability to accommodate a large amount of flow and dilatation). The placement of TIPS has become (increasingly) the treatment of choice for recurrent bleeding of such varices.

TABLE 8.1: **Etiology of Portal Hypertension**

Prehepatic (before or at the entrance to the liver), when the flow cannot properly enter the liver	**Hepatic** (inside the liver), when the flow from the portal system cannot efficiently reach the inferior vena cava (IVC)	**Posthepatic** (after or at the exit of the liver), when the flow cannot properly exit the liver through the IVC
Congenital narrowing (i.e., atresia) of portal vein(s), which will increase pressure proximal to the narrowing	Cirrhosis and resulting liver fibrosis	Occlusion of the IVC from primary or secondary tumor and subsequent thrombosis or from extrinsic compression
Thrombosis of portal veins (from different causes such as secondary tumor or cirrhosis)	Schistosomiasis, a parasitic infection resulting in damage to the liver parenchyma	Budd-Chiari syndrome, a condition characterized by thrombosed hepatic veins
Compression of portal vein(s) (from different etiologies such as masses, enlarged lymph nodes, etc.)	Chronic hepatitis, also resulting in damage to the liver parenchyma	Some cardiac anomalies that result in increased pressure in the right atrium (such as right-sided heart failure)
Arteriovenous malformations within the liver parenchyma (acquired from biopsies or congenital)	Tumors	
Thrombosis of the splenic vein (which could increase flow in the portal system)		
Enlargement of the spleen or splenomegaly (which could also increase flow in the portal system)		

Although the evaluation of TIPS by ultrasound is still relatively rare for multiple reasons that are beyond the scope of this book, understanding the findings before and after placement offers great educational and clinical opportunities.

Tips/Rationale

- TIPS procedure for:
  - Alleviating portal hypertension (mostly as a result of cirrhosis from alcoholism complications or viral infection such as hepatitis B) when significant esophageal or gastric varices are bleeding or have the potential for bleeding and/or when the bleeding is refractory to other treatment options.
  - Refractory ascites (sometimes), which is the accumulation of fluid within the peritoneal cavity.
- Complications:
  - TIPS stenosis (frequent), thrombosis, and infections
  - TIPS misplacement
  - Hepatic encephalopathy, which is also a complication of liver failure and portal hypertension, occurs when TIPS dysfunction fails to relieve portal hypertension within the first few days, but it also occurs as an almost unavoidable consequence of the procedure in the long term due to accumulation of nitrogenous compounds (from portal diversion to the systemic circulation).
  - Infarction can occur but it is very rare because in cirrhotic liver, although the portal vein supply may be decreased, it is compensated by an enlargement of the hepatic arteries supplying the liver tissue (and replacing the delivery of oxygen normally assumed at 70% by the portal veins).

Protocol Algorithm

Due to the nature of this chapter, debates about the role of ultrasound in the evaluation of TIPS, and the rarity of this exam in vascular laboratories, it is difficult to propose a protocol algorithm. In settings where these exams are performed more routinely, the evaluation by ultrasound may include a pre-TIPS exam, a post-TIPS exam (usually within 72 hours), and subsequent follow-ups at 3 and 6 months. It should be noted that in most setting, a venogram will almost invariably be added to the evaluation. The rationale is that venograms are the only exams allowing for pressure measurements (which cannot be done by ultrasound) within the TIPS with direct visualization of the cause of dysfunction and a route for immediate repair if needed.

Duplex Ultrasound Evaluation

Test Preparation

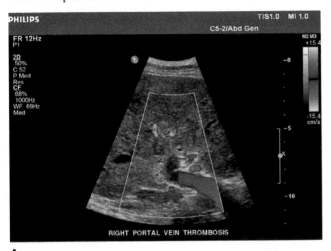

A

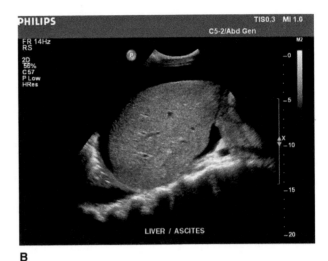

B

FIGURE 8.3. Examples of the causes of portal hypertension: portal vein thrombosis and liver cirrhosis with ascites.

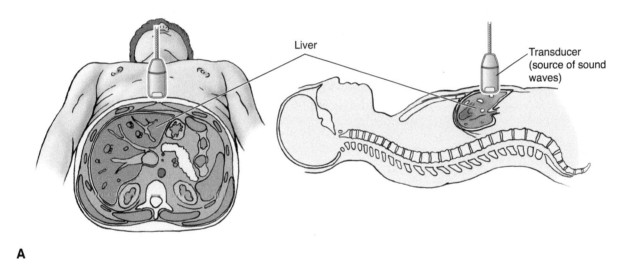

A

Liver

Transducer
(source of sound
waves)

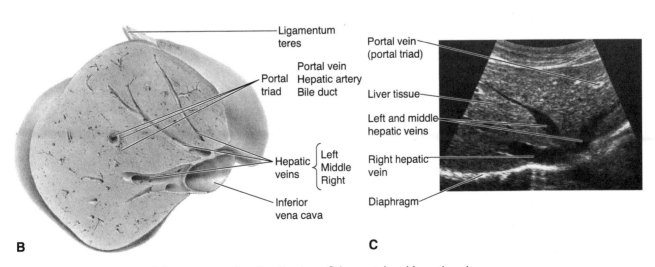

B

Ligamentum
teres

Portal
triad

Portal vein
Hepatic artery
Bile duct

Hepatic
veins

{
Left
Middle
Right

Inferior
vena cava

C

Portal vein
(portal triad)

Liver tissue

Left and middle
hepatic veins

Right hepatic
vein

Diaphragm

FIGURE 8.4. Diagrams of the sequence for visualization of the portal and hepatic veins.

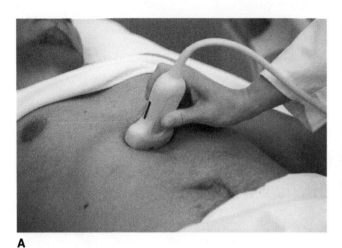 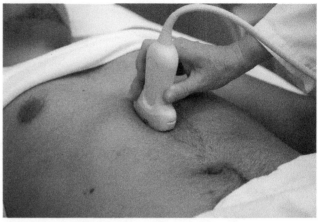

A   **B**

FIGURE 8.5.   Approach for beginning the evaluation of the portal veins, the hepatic artery, and the hepatic veins. The transducer will follow the rib cage margin and its orientation will shift from a transverse to longitudinal or sagittal orientation for each vessel as needed.

Testing Sequence

As expressed earlier, the goal of this chapter is slightly different than that of previous chapters. The testing sequence will, more than for any routine exams in vascular laboratories, be directed by the protocols in use in particular laboratory settings and the conditions of the patients. However, it is strongly recommended that certain elements (see Table 8.2) be present as described by the Intersocietal Commission for the Accreditation of Vascular Laboratories (ICAVL).

TABLE 8.2: Minimum Recommendations for Evaluation of Hepatoportal Circulation

General and Pre-TIPS Evaluation	Post-TIPS Evaluation
Intrahepatic portal veins (right and left) in B mode and Doppler	Collaterals in B mode and Doppler
Extrahepatic portal vein (main) in B mode and Doppler	Portal vein inflow in B mode and Doppler
Hepatic veins (right, left, and middle) in B mode and Doppler	Portal end of the stent in B mode and Doppler
Inferior vena cava in B mode and Doppler	Mid-stent in B mode and Doppler
Liver parenchyma in B mode	Hepatic end of the stent in B mode and Doppler
Collateral pathways and/or portosystemic shunts (if present) with Doppler	Hepatic vein outflow in B mode and Doppler
Spleen and splenic vein and superior mesenteric vein in B mode and Doppler	

Note: With Doppler (color and/or pulsed wave), one should note precisely the direction of flow in each vessel, as well as the velocities and characteristics of the waveforms obtained.

Results and Interpretation

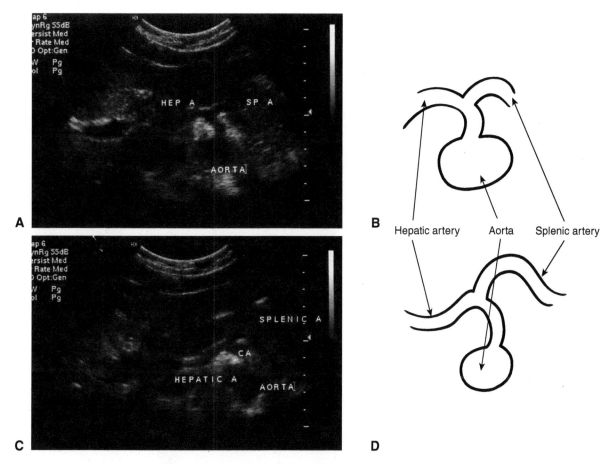

FIGURE 8.6.   Origin of the common hepatic artery. Note: At this level, the hepatic artery is called the common hepatic artery. At the level of the porta hepatis, the common hepatic artery is referred to as the proper hepatic artery. The proper hepatic artery contributes approximately 30% of the flow to the liver. The remaining 70% is contributed by the main portal vein.

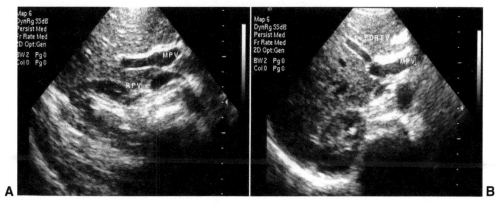

FIGURE 8.7.   Position of the main, right, and left portal veins. The portal veins are usually characterized by bright walls. The main portal vein (formed by the confluence of the superior mesenteric vein and splenic vein, which has received flow from the inferior mesenteric vein) divides, shortly after entry into the inferior portion of the liver at the porta hepatis, into the right and left portal veins. The veins will divide further to enter each segment of the liver (they are intrasegmental). Their orientation is, in general, "horizontal," so transverse or slightly oblique views allow for visualization of the length of the vessels.

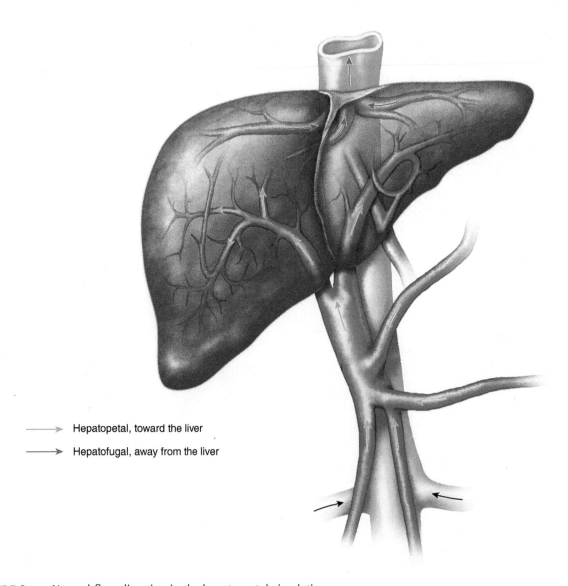

FIGURE 8.8.   Position of the right, left, and middle hepatic veins. The hepatic veins have thin walls with poorly discernible margins. These veins are intersegmental in the liver (and run within liver fissures). They are the main port of egress from the liver (at the superior portion) to the systemic circulation in the inferior vena cava. They typically enlarge as they approach the inferior vena cava (IVC). They do not contain valves. Their orientation is, in general, "vertical," forming a three-dimensional grid with the portal vein branches. Sagittal views allow for visualization of the length of the vessels.

Hepatopetal, toward the liver

Hepatofugal, away from the liver

FIGURE 8.9.   Normal flow direction in the hepatoportal circulation.

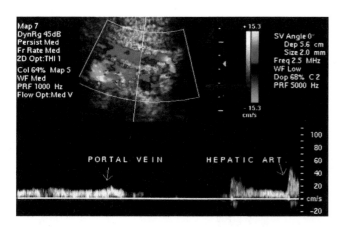

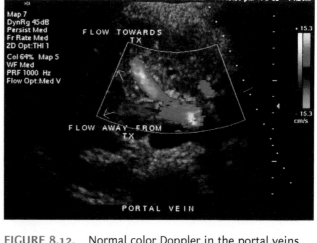

FIGURE 8.10. Normal flow direction in the main portal vein and proper hepatic artery at entrance in the liver at the porta hepatis. The portal vein has slightly undulating flow (which increases with digestion), and the hepatic artery demonstrates low-resistance flow (which may slightly decrease with digestion to accommodate the increased flow from the portal vein).

FIGURE 8.12. Normal color Doppler in the portal veins.

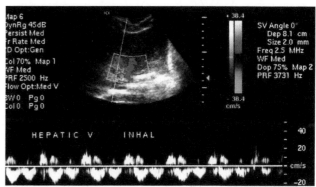

FIGURE 8.13. Normal color and pulsed wave (PW) Doppler in the hepatic veins. Due to the proximity of the inferior vena cava (IVC) and the right atrium of the heart, the hepatic veins should demonstrate rather pulsatile Doppler waveforms. Important interpretation point: In this image, the color spectrum was stopped during the "reverse" phase, actually displaying here a hepatopetal flow. However, the PW Doppler waveforms clearly demonstrate hepatofugal flow.

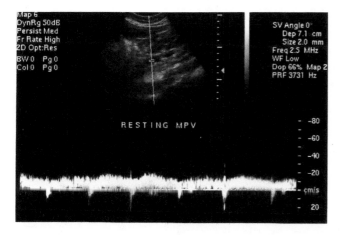

FIGURE 8.11. Normal Doppler waveforms in the main portal vein.

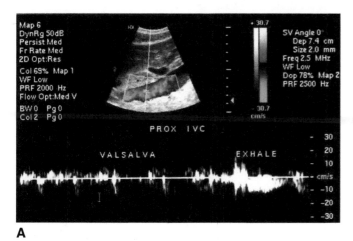

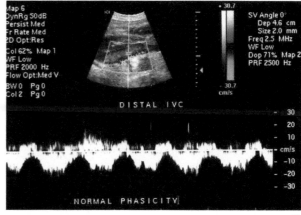

A

B

FIGURE 8.14. Normal color and pulsed wave Doppler in the inferior vena.

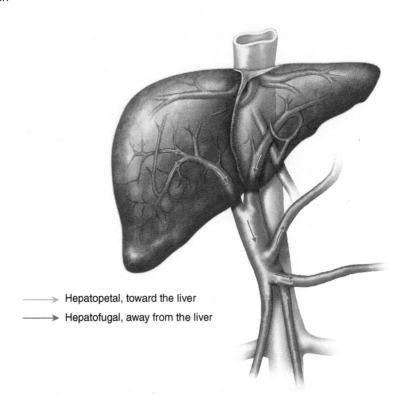

Hepatopetal, toward the liver

Hepatofugal, away from the liver

FIGURE 8.15. Sample of flow patterns with portal hypertension: reversal of flow in portal veins shunting through coronary veins or other routes, leading to varices.

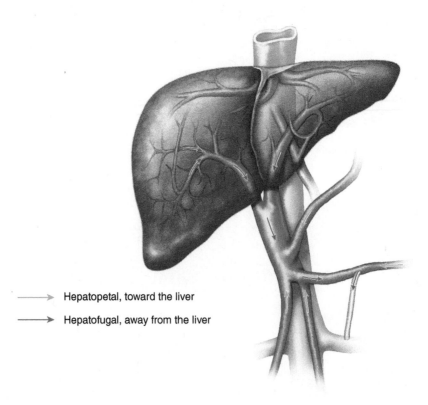

Hepatopetal, toward the liver

Hepatofugal, away from the liver

FIGURE 8.16. Sample of flow patterns with portal hypertension: spontaneous splenorenal shunt.

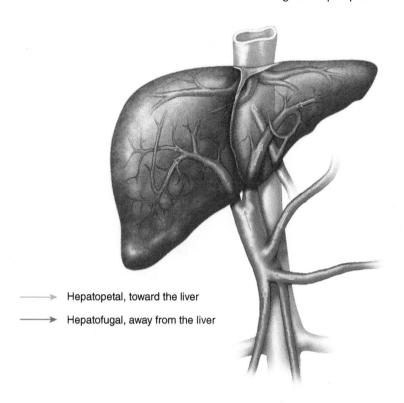

FIGURE 8.17.   Sample of flow patterns with portal hypertension: recanalization of paraumbilical vein leading to dilatation of abdominal superficial veins, caput medusae.

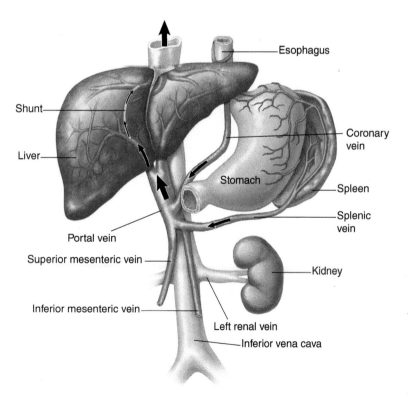

FIGURE 8.18.   TIPS implantation and flow direction.

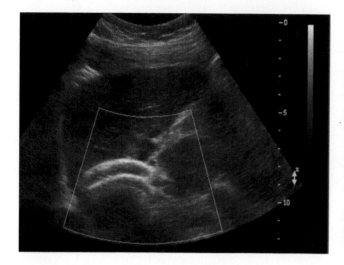

FIGURE 8.19. Main body of TIPS (close to portal end).

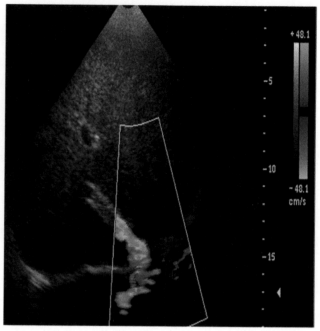

FIGURE 8.20. Hepatic end of TIPS.

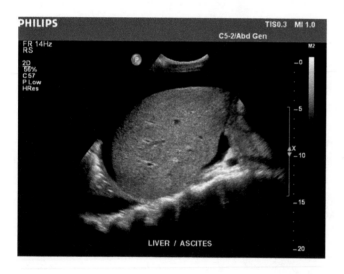

FIGURE 8.21. Ascites. Courtesy of Philips.

TABLE 8.3: **Findings after TIPS**

	TIPS	Portal Veins (PVs)	Hepatic Veins
Flow direction	Hepatopetal and portal end, and toward inferior vena cava (IVC) at hepatic end	Flow in the left PV and anterior branch of right PV toward TIPS (hepatofugal)	No change, i.e., toward IVC
Velocities	High velocities, usually > 90 cm/s and up to 200 cm/s, turbulent flow (due to direct connection with systemic circulation)	Velocities < 50 cm/s at the portal end of the TIPS suggest stenosis within the TIPS	
Other findings	Stenosis in the TIPS will also be suggested with findings of new onset of ascites or recurrent varices.	Caution: if the patient has a well-recanalized umbilical vein, the blood will continue to divert out of the liver, and the flow in the left portal vein will continue to be hepatopetal despite a well-functioning shunt!!	When stenosis is present, flow may reverse and be directed toward the TIPS.

Concluding Tips

The liver vasculature in the normal state requires a thorough understanding of the anatomy and physiology and a great attention to detail, particularly of flow direction, but this can be easily mastered. In disease, such as with portal hypertension, the challenges can be overcome if:

- You are comfortable with your understanding of normal anatomy and physiology.

- You understand the concepts of hemodynamics and remember primarily that flow will always take the path of least resistance.

- You keep a very detailed atlas of anatomy handy to foresee possible collateral pathways.

- You keep a thorough documentation of the flow direction observed in vessels you may not normally see, as well as those that would obviously be involved in the pathologic process. This point is particularly important when performing evaluation after TIPS because sudden changes in flow direction from previous exams are great indirect indicators of poor functioning.

- You keep an open mind about the different possibilities for collateral pathways. Varices have been documented in the vessels of the gall bladder (the cystic vein is a branch of the portal vein too!) and in the paravertebral space, and spontaneous shunt can develop between the splenic vein and left renal veins.

References

Owens, C. A., Bartolone, C., Warner, D. L., et al. (1998). The inaccuracy of duplex ultrasonography in predicting patency of TIPS. *Gastroenterology, 114*, 975–980.

Carr, C. E., Tuite, C. M., Soulen, M. C., et al. (2006). Role of ultrasound surveillance of TIPS in the covered stent era. *Journal of Vascular Interventional Radiology, 17*, 1297–1305.

CHAPTER 9

PART FOUR: PELVIS AND LOWER EXTREMITIES

Testing the Arterial Circulation

Chapter Outline

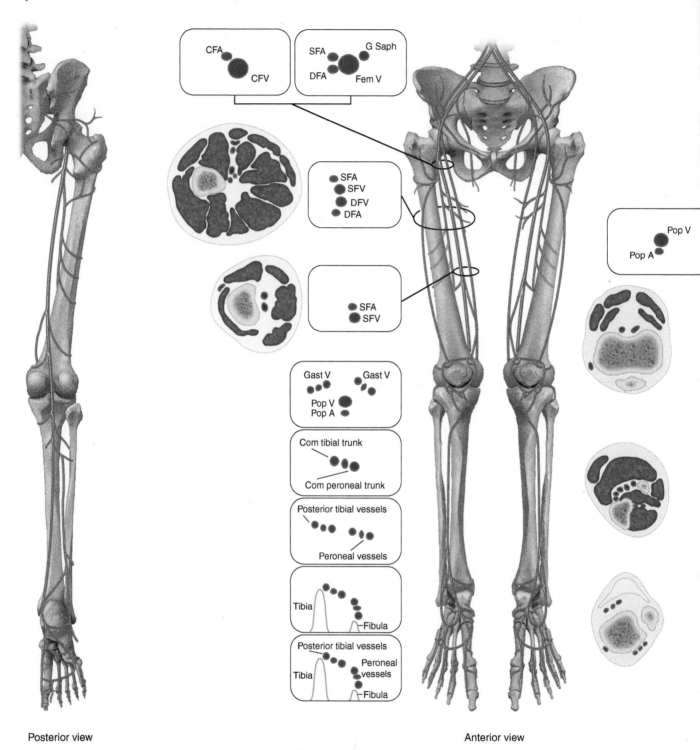

FIGURE 9.1.   Diagrams of arteries of lower extremities (anterior and posterior view).

General Concepts in Arterial Circulation Examination

Tips/Rationale

The underlying rationale for uncovering and reporting information through a diagnostic test should always be linked to what is available for either preventing further problems or for alleviating the symptoms tied to the condition. Advances in the treatment of arterial diseases, through bypass graft, angioplasty and stent, endarterectomy, medication, and even prosthesis for limb replacement, have rendered the role of diagnostic imaging and, in particular, ultrasound vascular laboratories central to any clinical vascular practice.

Without entering too deep into the existential or philosophical arena, it seems that for bipedal human beings, retaining the full use of lower limbs is paramount for self-esteem, integrity, and functionality. Testing the arterial circulation of the lower extremities should therefore include a thorough understanding not only of the patient's underlying condition or cause for the condition, but also and more importantly the patient's lifestyle and desired level of functionality.

With arterial disease, independent of the underlying pathology, there will be a restriction of blood flow to an organ or tissue. The role of the sonographer will be to determine:

1. If the symptoms are truly due to a restriction of flow,
2. Where the restriction of flow is, and
3. How severe the restriction of flow is.

In this chapter, this will pertain to the lower extremities and therefore the function of the skeletal muscles of the thigh and leg and their roles in ambulation. Because it is a matter of function, a baseline test should always be a physiologic test, which will answer question 1. Duplex scanning and transcutaneous oxygen pressure are other testing modalities that can be useful in answering questions 2 and 3.

Keep in mind that there may be additional conditions either limiting the value of the baseline test and/or mimicking arterial pathology. Reconciling the test results to the history and symptoms will add valuable information in unraveling the weight of each factor and determining the best route for follow-up or treatment.

Protocol Algorithms

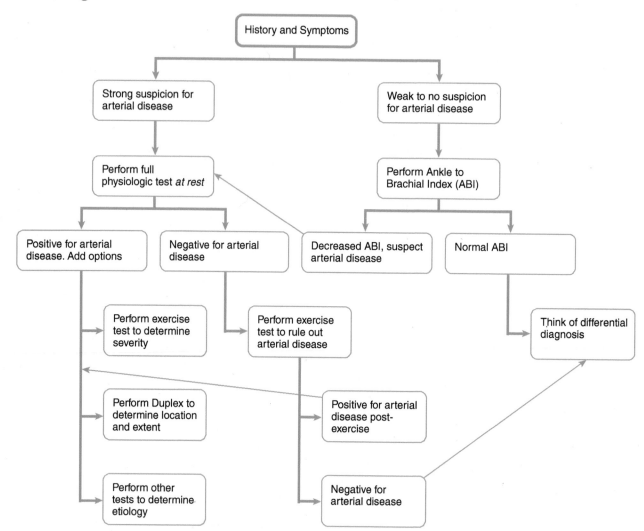

FIGURE 9.2. Recommended algorithm for testing the arterial circulation of the lower extremities in accordance with the following three questions: (1) Are the symptoms truly due to a restriction of flow? (2) Where is the restriction of flow? (3) How severe is the restriction of flow?

Physiologic Studies

Tips/Rationale

- Patient and sonographer comfort is crucial for a successful exam, mostly because cold, stress, and position will affect hemodynamics.
- Explain the procedure. Do not minimize the possibility of discomfort mostly from the pressure from the cuffs or underestimate the time needed for the test, particularly if you need to proceed with exercise.
- Assist the patient when needed with changing into the gown and with positioning on the examination table.
- Keep the room at a temperature comfortable for the patient (75°F), and cover parts that do not need to be exposed at all time (provide socks and a blanket).
- Patient should be supine with arms and legs in the same horizontal plane as the heart. The head can be slightly elevated for comfort.

- The tests should always be performed first at rest (you should always allow the patient to rest for at least 10 to 15 minutes before proceeding with the exam; this time will be efficiently filled by obtaining the patient's information, helping the patient, and preparing for the test).

- Wash your hands and disinfect the Doppler tip (doing this in front of the patient will increase his or her comfort in the quality of the exam and the facility). Clean cuffs as needed (but at least once a day).

- Proceed with preparing all you will need for the test. Because this test is concerned with the hemodynamics of the arterial tree in regard to the physiology of the tissue supplied, it is essential that your time management be consistent with potential physiologic changes (comfort, warmth, stress level, pain and discomfort, exercise timing, etc.)

Test Preparation

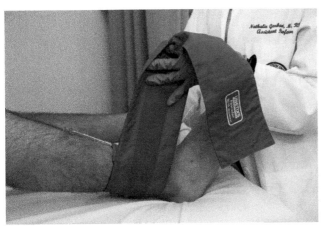

A

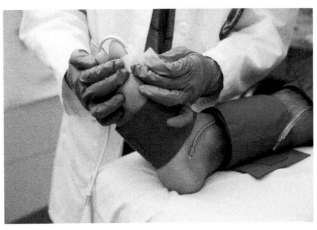

B

FIGURE 9.3.   Placing cuffs. This step is essential for obtaining adequate data but also for time management. Two tests will be dependent on the accurate placement of cuffs. Placing extra cuffs at the metatarsal level and toe can be considered for an extended test and/or additional information.

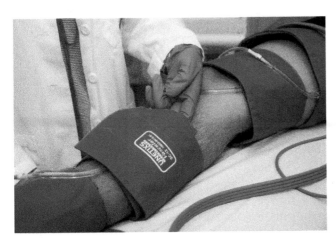

FIGURE 9.4.   As already mentioned, the accurate placement of cuffs is essential for several tests. Here the sonographer tests the snugness of the cuffs.

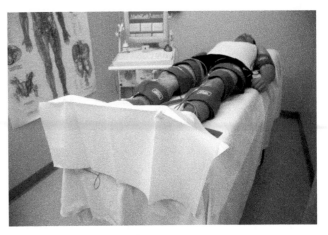

FIGURE 9.5.   The patient is ready for the start of the test. Ensure the patient is comfortable by slightly elevating the head and warming the feet with a blanket or towel.

Testing Sequence

■ A <u>complete</u> physiologic test should include at a minimum:

- Pulse volume recording (PVR) at the high thigh, low thigh, below knee, and ankle levels. Metatarsal and toe are strongly recommended for a baseline, but may also be added for completeness or based on symptoms. However, it is often better to have too much information at baseline than having to add or repeat a step after an already long exam.

- Segmental pressures at the same minimum levels as PVR (i.e., high thigh, low thigh, below knee, and ankle). Toe pressures usually do not need to be added unless more proximal vessels were found to be non-compressible.

- Continuous wave Doppler waveforms at the common femoral, mid superficial femoral, popliteal, anterior tibial/dorsalis pedis, and posterior tibial arteries. The peroneal artery should be included when either of the other two tibial arteries cannot be assessed.

- All steps should be done on both limbs, except of course in case of amputation. However, evaluating the stump of an amputated leg with PVR and Doppler may provide valuable information for follow-up.

■ Additional physiologic tests are:

- Photoplethysmography (PPG), which would be used if small arteries of the digit are felt to be involved in the disease process.

- Transcutaneous oxygen pressure ($TcPO_2$), which would be used to evaluate further the potential for the healing of an ulcer by itself or through intervention, as with hyperbaric oxygen treatment, or to determine the most appropriate level for amputation.

Proximal

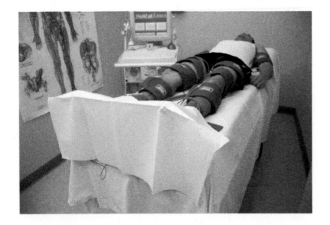 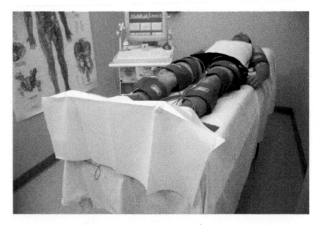

Distal

FIGURE 9.6. The sequence of inflation of cuffs for PVR should be from the most distal to the most proximal. The rationale for this sequencing is to avoid creating reactive hyperemia. Indeed, even though the cuffs are only inflated to 65 mmHg, repeated inflation from proximal to distal may by itself mimic increased metabolic demand and compensation seen with disease.

FIGURE 9.7. The sequence of inflation of cuffs for segmental pressures start at the brachial level (point of reference) and proceed to the lower extremities in a similar fashion (with same rationale) as with PVR. The main differences are that: (1) the cuffs will be inflated to suprasystolic pressure at all levels and (2) pressures will be taken at the ankle, listening at the anterior and the posterior tibial arteries.

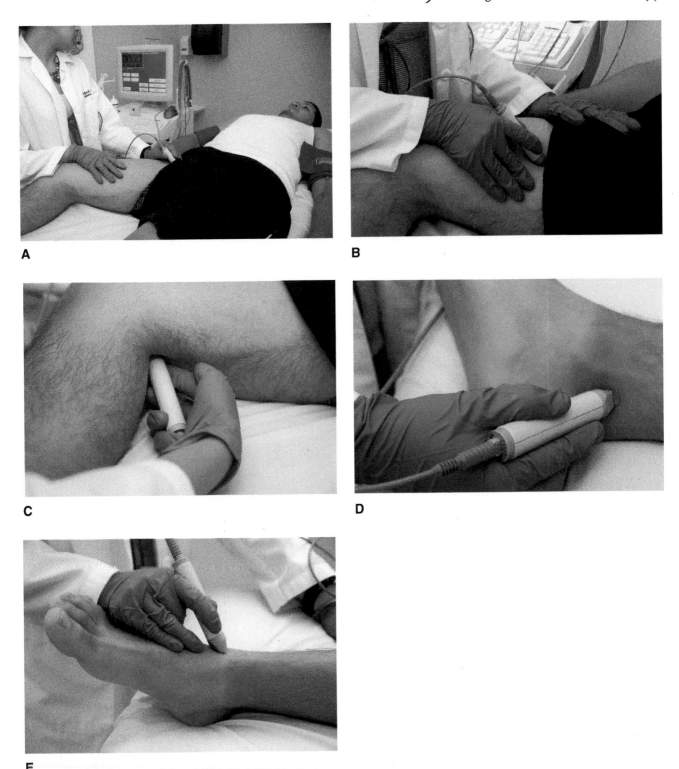

FIGURE 9.8. The sequence for obtaining continuous wave (CW) Doppler waveforms can be tailored to the comfort and preference of the sonographer; unlike any of the tests involving cuffs, there is no special consideration or rationale for using one sequence over another. However, an effort should be made to obtain waveforms at all predetermined levels with a correct position (as shown) on the pencil probe in relation to the artery: (A) at the common femoral artery (CFA); (B) at the superficial femoral artery (SFA); (C) at the popliteal artery; (D) at the posterior tibial artery (PTA); and (E) at the anterior tibial artery (ATA) distally.

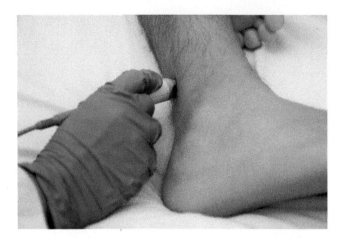

FIGURE 9.9.   The peroneal artery is usually not included in a typical exam. However, it can be an alternate site to listen for Doppler signal for ankle pressure and can give additional information about foot perfusion.

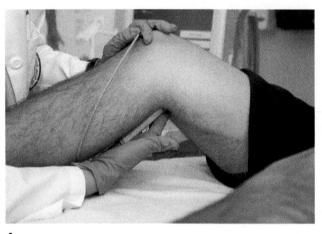

A

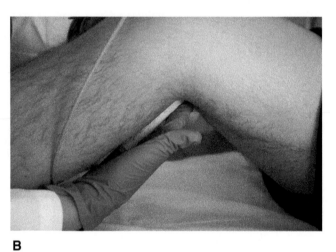

B

FIGURE 9.10.   This position is an alternate to obtaining continuous wave (CW) Doppler waveform at the popliteal artery. Aim for the mid-popliteal fossa with the pencil probe resting against the belly of the calf to ensure proper angle.

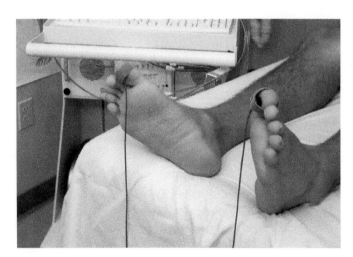

FIGURE 9.11.   PPG leads are a great modality to obtain toe pressure. The leads should be placed over the "fleshy" part of the digit and secured (not too tight) with Velcro, double-sided tape, or surgical cloth tape (take into consideration possible allergic reaction to tape).

Results and Interpretation

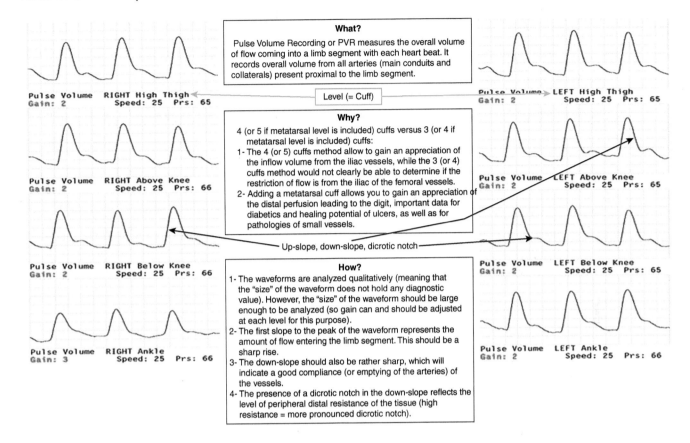

What?

Pulse Volume Recording or PVR measures the overall volume of flow coming into a limb segment with each heart beat. It records overall volume from all arteries (main conduits and collaterals) present proximal to the limb segment.

Level (= Cuff)

Why?

4 (or 5 if metatarsal level is included) cuffs versus 3 (or 4 if metatarsal level is included) cuffs:

1- The 4 (or 5) cuffs method allow to gain an appreciation of the inflow volume from the iliac vessels, while the 3 (or 4) cuffs method would not clearly be able to determine if the restriction of flow is from the iliac of the femoral vessels.

2- Adding a metatarsal cuff allows you to gain an appreciation of the distal perfusion leading to the digit, important data for diabetics and healing potential of ulcers, as well as for pathologies of small vessels.

Up-slope, down-slope, dicrotic notch

How?

1- The waveforms are analyzed qualitatively (meaning that the "size" of the waveform does not hold any diagnostic value). However, the "size" of the waveform should be large enough to be analyzed (so gain can and should be adjusted at each level for this purpose).

2- The first slope to the peak of the waveform represents the amount of flow entering the limb segment. This should be a sharp rise.

3- The down-slope should also be rather sharp, which will indicate a good compliance (or emptying of the arteries) of the vessels.

4- The presence of a dicrotic notch in the down-slope reflects the level of peripheral distal resistance of the tissue (high resistance = more pronounced dicrotic notch).

Pulse Volume RIGHT High Thigh
Gain: 2   Speed: 25 Prs: 65

Pulse Volume RIGHT Above Knee
Gain: 2   Speed: 25 Prs: 66

Pulse Volume RIGHT Below Knee
Gain: 2   Speed: 25 Prs: 66

Pulse Volume RIGHT Ankle
Gain: 3   Speed: 25 Prs: 66

Pulse Volume LEFT High Thigh
Gain: 2   Speed: 25 Prs: 65

Pulse Volume LEFT Above Knee
Gain: 2   Speed: 25 Prs: 65

Pulse Volume LEFT Below Knee
Gain: 2   Speed: 25 Prs: 65

Pulse Volume LEFT Ankle
Gain: 2   Speed: 25 Prs: 66

FIGURE 9.12.   PVR essential tips.

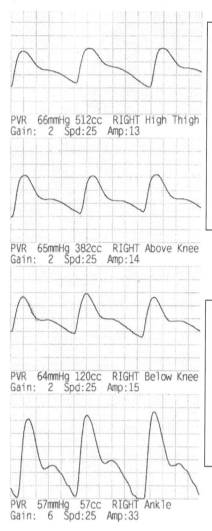

PVR 66mmHg 512cc RIGHT High Thigh
Gain: 2 Spd:25 Amp:13

PVR 65mmHg 382cc RIGHT Above Knee
Gain: 2 Spd:25 Amp:14

PVR 64mmHg 120cc RIGHT Below Knee
Gain: 2 Spd:25 Amp:15

PVR 57mmHg 57cc RIGHT Ankle
Gain: 6 Spd:25 Amp:33

Point 1:
This piece of equipment includes the volume of air added to each cuff to attain the set pressure. Since most tests will be performed on both lower extremities simultaneously, using the same size cuff for each level, and assuming a relative symmetry in size at each segment, the volume of air should be similar. The following rule of thumb can be applied:

A- < 100 cc difference for the high thigh level

B- between 20 and 50 cc difference for all other levels

Considering at all time the limb size and the cuff size.

In this case > 100 cc difference at the thigh level may tip the sonographer that the right high thigh cuff may have a looser fit than the left. Although it does not affect the results here because the flow is normal, this may render the analysis of the waveforms more difficult when disease is present.

Point 2:
Note the size of the waveforms and the gain used to obtain each waveform. Although as previously noted the "size" itself does not enter into the diagnostic value of the waveform, it is important that waveforms at each level can be correctly analyzed.

Because at the thigh level the flow is mostly delivered to the segment through 2 main arteries, the superficial and deep femoral arteries, for a relatively large mass of muscles, compared to the calf where 3 arteries supply the segment for a considerably smaller muscle mass, the deflection with PVR will be different. To compensate, the gain should be increased at the thigh. This is mostly a matter of ease of analysis and again does not have any diagnostic values.

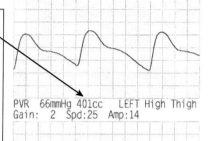
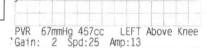
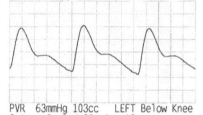
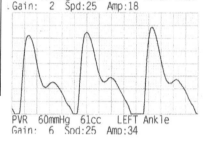
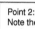

PVR 66mmHg 401cc   LEFT High Thigh
Gain: 2 Spd:25 Amp:14

PVR 67mmHg 457cc   LEFT Above Knee
Gain: 2 Spd:25 Amp:13

PVR 63mmHg 103cc   LEFT Below Knee
Gain: 2 Spd:25 Amp:18

PVR 60mmHg 61cc   LEFT Ankle
Gain: 6 Spd:25 Amp:34

FIGURE 9.13.   Cautions in PVR analysis.

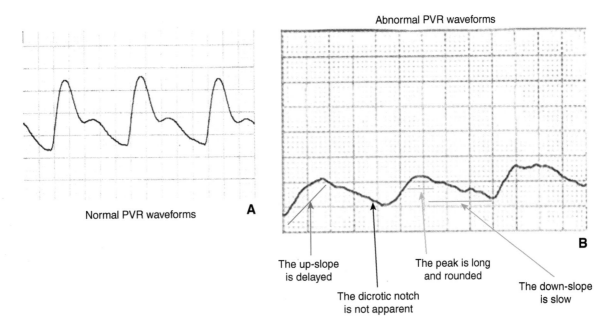

Abnormal PVR waveforms

Normal PVR waveforms   **A**

B

The up-slope
is delayed

The peak is long
and rounded

The dicrotic notch
is not apparent

The down-slope
is slow

FIGURE 9.14. Sample of normal (A) and abnormal (B) PVR. What does it mean? (1) The flow getting to this segment of the limb is delayed. This could be from a severe stenosis proximal to the segment or from an occlusion proximal to the segment with flow supplied by small collaterals. (2) The disease may be long standing and/or disseminated. The disappearance of the dicrotic notch particularly indicates vasodilation of the arteries in distal segment. (3) A complete evaluation of the level of disease can only be performed with analysis of sequential waveforms from both lower extremities to assess the change between segments.

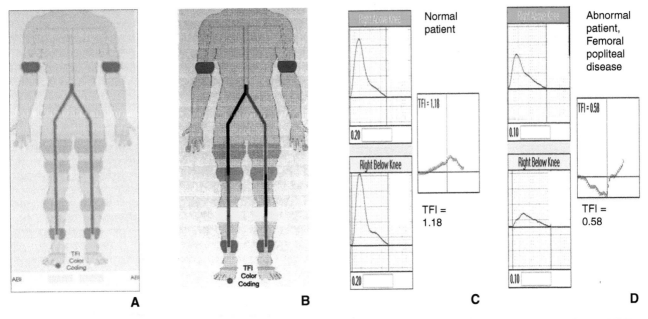

Normal patient

Right Above Knee

TFI = 1.18

Right Below Knee

TFI = 1.18

Abnormal patient, Femoral popliteal disease

Right Above Knee

TFI = 0.58

Right Below Knee

TFI = 0.58

A   **B**   **C**   **D**

FIGURE 9.15. New application for PVR, transfer function index (TFI). TFI is only available on equipment from Nicolet. This technique offers ease of use and accuracy in the diagnosis of stenosis and occlusion within the peripheral arterial tree, yet it has not found widespread utilization. The concept is based on a computed averaging ($>$ 30 to 40 cardiac cycles) of the amplitude of standard PVR waveforms between inflow and outflow. In a simple, limited test, PVRs at the brachial and ankle levels are taken simultaneously, and the software computes the TFI. The TFI is expressed as a number (as shown in the figure) and has been correlated as follows: $>$ 0.90 (mean = 1.05) usually represents no significant disease between two sites, approximately 0.72 represents stenosis, and $<$ 0.67 correlates with occlusion. The concept can be applied to multiple segments (with one cuff at the thigh level) and computed to inflow/outflow sequentially. The results are displayed with the TFI as well as color coding of arterial segments representing degrees of severity of disease (red = normal, blue = mild to moderate, and black = severe to occlusion). The results have shown a very strong correlation with angiographic and duplex ultrasound results.

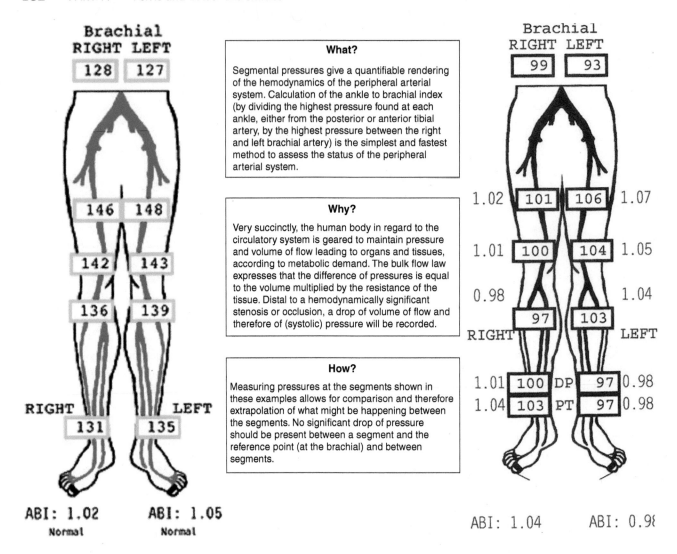

Brachial

RIGHT	LEFT
128	127

146	148
142	143
136	139

RIGHT   LEFT

| 131 | 135 |

ABI: 1.02   ABI: 1.05
Normal   Normal

What?

Segmental pressures give a quantifiable rendering of the hemodynamics of the peripheral arterial system. Calculation of the ankle to brachial index (by dividing the highest pressure found at each ankle, either from the posterior or anterior tibial artery, by the highest pressure between the right and left brachial artery) is the simplest and fastest method to assess the status of the peripheral arterial system.

Why?

Very succinctly, the human body in regard to the circulatory system is geared to maintain pressure and volume of flow leading to organs and tissues, according to metabolic demand. The bulk flow law expresses that the difference of pressures is equal to the volume multiplied by the resistance of the tissue. Distal to a hemodynamically significant stenosis or occlusion, a drop of volume of flow and therefore of (systolic) pressure will be recorded.

How?

Measuring pressures at the segments shown in these examples allows for comparison and therefore extrapolation of what might be happening between the segments. No significant drop of pressure should be present between a segment and the reference point (at the brachial) and between segments.

Brachial

RIGHT	LEFT
99	93

1.02	101	106	1.07
1.01	100	104	1.05
0.98	97	103	1.04

RIGHT   LEFT

| 1.01 | 100 | DP | 97 | 0.98 |
| 1.04 | 103 | PT | 97 | 0.98 |

ABI: 1.04   ABI: 0.98

FIGURE 9.16.   Essential tips regarding segmental pressures.

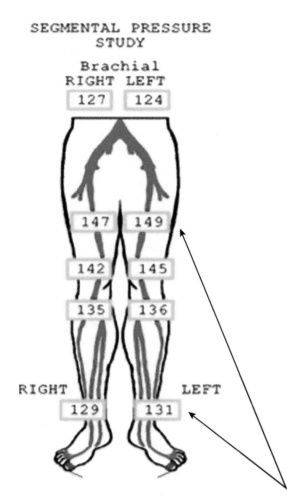

SEGMENTAL PRESSURE
STUDY

Brachial
RIGHT LEFT
127   124

147   149

142   145

135   136

RIGHT   LEFT
129   131

ABI: 1.02   ABI: 1.03

FIGURE 9.17.   Cautions in segmental pressures analysis.

Interpreting Pressure:

• A 20 mmHg drop in pressure is usually linked to hemodynamically significant disease

• However, cuffs used for evaluation of pressures in adult limbs are manufactured mainly in two bladder sizes: 12 cm and 10 cm

• The American Heart Association recommends that a cuff be 80% of the length and 40% of the width of the limb segment

• At the high thigh cuff level, particularly, and with the limitation of cuff sizes available, even a 12 cm cuff bladder may be too narrow

• This will result in a artifactually high pressure at the thigh, usually in the order of 20 to 30 mmHg

• When compared to other segments (which may be more appropriate for the size of the cuff used), it may appear that a significant drop has occurred even when no disease is present

• Calcified vessels (such as the tibial arteries in diabetes) will usually not be compressible at tolerable systolic pressure (up to 240-250 mmHg). These pressure recordings should be discounted as they are diagnostically invalid

• The Vascular Disease Foundation recommend that any ABI>1.3 be deemed invalid for diagnostic purposes (as they would likely be linked to erroneously high pressures at the ankle from noncompressible vessels)

Relative difference in pressures

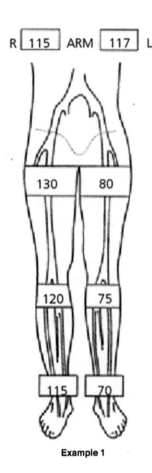

Tip 1:
Analyze pressure drop from point of reference, i.e., brachial pressure (representing the "estimated" central pressure)

Tip 2:
Do not forget to consider limb and cuff size. In example 1 the thigh pressure is higher, which may be due to slightly inappropriate cuff size

Tip 3:
Analyze pressure results from side to side at the same level and from proximal to distal segment in the same limb

Example 1:
There is a drop between the central pressure and the left high thigh, but no additional drop. However, the right high thigh has expected pressure value. This would lead the sonographer to believe that a significant lesion might be present in the left iliac arterial system.

Example 2:
There is a drop of pressure between the right thigh and below knee cuff (36 mmHg), as well as between the left below knee ankle cuff (67 mmHg). Since the size of the limb is not known a difference a drop of 36 mmHg may represent only mild disease within the right femoral system. A drop of 67 mmHg on the left leg represents most likely a very severe stenosis or occlusion of one of the tibial vessels (taking two ankle pressures may let you make that distinction).

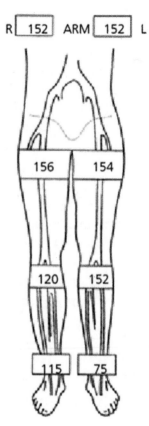

Example 1

Example 2

FIGURE 9.18.   Samples of abnormal segmental pressure sequences.

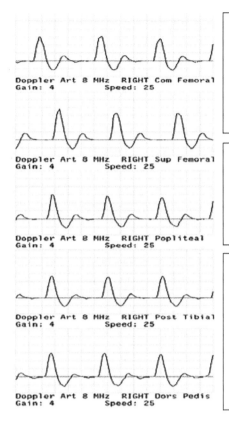

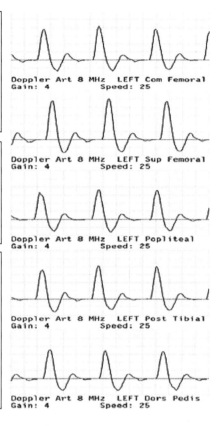

What?

The continuous wave Doppler waveform is a representation of the changes of frequency shifts, flow velocities, and ultimately the energy waves variations throughout a cardiac cycle. The amount of flow during the pulse wave, as well as the compliance of the vessel and the distal resistance of the tissues, all play an important role in the quality or shape of the waveform.

Why?

Unlike PVR waveforms and segmental pressure measurements to some extent, the CW Doppler waveforms allow for a more directed analysis of a particular vessel, i.e., the one being insonated (even though CW Doppler does not allow to truly distinguish the vessel in the path of the ultrasound beam).

How?

Although we are not recording velocities with CW Doppler waveforms, the angle of insonation of the pencil probe to the direction of the vessel is important (as underlined in the next figure). CW waveforms are as PVR waveforms analyzed qualitatively. A normal waveform should have a sharp upstroke in systole, some reverse component in diastole, followed by a slight forward component in late diastole (representing the compliance of the vessels through the rebound of the arterial wall from the stored energy).

FIGURE 9.19.   Continuous wave Doppler essential tips.

Technical Error 1:
This waveform accounts for some of the limitation of CW Doppler, where all vessels in the path of the ultrasound are recorded (making the diastolic component difficult to interpret). Isolating a single vessel is rather tricky but great care should be put to do so.

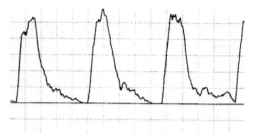

Dop 8Mhz   LEFT Common Femoral
Gain: 32 Hz/mm   Speed:25

Technical Error 2:
This waveform is most likely the result of a poor angle of the Doppler probe in relation to the artery. Applying too much pressure at the site on insonation with the pencil probe onto the artery may also result in such a waveform where the diastolic component is not visible.

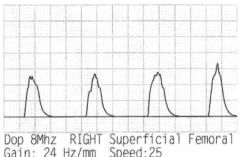

Dop 8Mhz   RIGHT Superficial Femoral
Gain: 24 Hz/mm   Speed:25

Technical Error 3:
Similar considerations as #2.

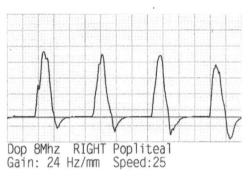

Dop 8Mhz   RIGHT Popliteal
Gain: 24 Hz/mm   Speed:25

FIGURE 9.20. Cautions in continuous wave (CW) Doppler waveforms analysis. All of the CW Doppler waveforms in this figure were taken from arteries without any evidence of pathology. The main message here is that it is rather easy (when not careful) to introduce errors in the CW Doppler waveform that can mimic disease (although it would be impossible to make an abnormal waveform look normal).

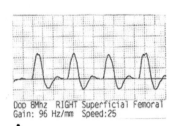

Dop 8Mhz   RIGHT Superficial Femoral
Gain: 96 Hz/mm   Speed:25

A

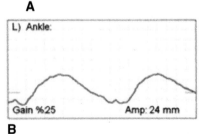

L) Ankle:

Gain %25   Amp: 24 mm

B

FIGURE 9.21. Samples of abnormal continuous wave (CW) Doppler waveforms.

Exercise Pressure Measurement											
	Rest	1	2	3	4	5	6	7	8	9	10
R Ankle (DP):	142	95	105	115	121	130	142				
L Ankle (DP):	144	145	145	143	144	144	144				
L Brachial:	142	158	154	150	145	142	142				
R ABI	1.00	0.60	0.68	0.77	0.83	0.92	1.00				
L ABI	1.01	0.92	0.94	0.95	0.99	1.01	1.01				

A

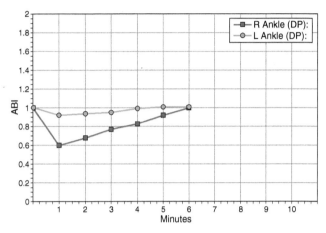

B

FIGURE 9.22. Postexercise pressure sequence example 1. This example shows two representations of the pressure and ankle-brachial index (ABI) values obtained after exercise. A significant decrease was noted in the right leg, and the sequence shows that it took 6 minutes for the ABI to return to resting value. A slight decrease was noted in the left leg with a return to resting value within 5 minutes. These results by themselves imply greater functionally limiting disease on the right. Pressure measurements could have been stopped at 5 minutes on the left.

RIGHT POST EXERCISE			
PER	BRA.	ANK.	ABI
Res	99	103	1.04
Imm	104	85	0.82
1	102	93	0.91
2	100	96	0.96
3			

LEFT POST EXERCISE			
PER	BRA.	ANK.	ABI
Res	99	97	0.98
Imm	104	89	0.86
1	102	94	0.92
2	100	90	0.90
3			

A   **B**

FIGURE 9.23. Postexercise pressure sequence example 2. A decrease in pressures at both ankles and ABI is noted here. Sequential measurements were taken at specified time interval (usually between 1 and 2 minutes). The main concern here is that the sonographer stopped at period 3, even though the ABIs were not back to resting values. Unless period 3 represents a 10-minute interval from the end of the exercise (the point we consider significant for the duration of symptoms), great care should be taken to continue taking pressures until the resting ABI values are reached.

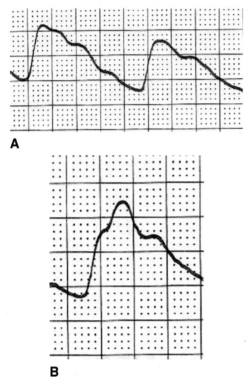

A

B

FIGURE 9.24.   PPG essentials. (A) Normal PPG of digit. As with PVR, PPG waveforms are analyzed quantitatively (refer to PVR for analysis). The amplitude of the waveform by itself does not hold much, if any, diagnostic value. (B) Abnormal PPG of digit. This waveform represents a typical waveform seen with Raynaud's disease or other vasospastic phenomenon.

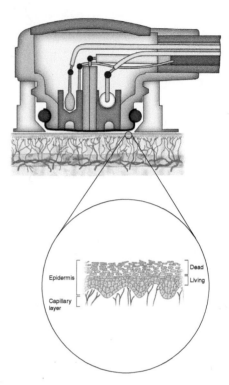

FIGURE 9.25.   Diagram of TcPO$_2$.

TABLE 9.1 Transcutaneous Oxygen Pressure (TcPO$_2$) Essentials

Ambient Pressure (ATA)/ Breathing Media	1.0 Air	1.0 O$_2$	2.0 O$_2$	2.4 O$_2$	3.0 O$_2$
Ambient PO$_2$, mmHg	159	760	1520	1824	2280
Transcutaneous PO$_2$ (mean all sites)	69 ± 6	440 ± 95		1350 ± 220	
Transcutaneous PO$_2$ – chest	67 ± 12	450 ± 54		1312 ± 112	
Transcutaneous PO$_2$ – calf, male	49 ± 14	281 ± 78		1027 ± 164	
Transcutaneous PO$_2$ – calf, female	59 ± 12	367 ± 59		1174 ± 127	
Transcutaneous PO$_2$ – midfoot	63 ± 13	280 ± 82		919 ± 214	
Transcutaneous PO$_2$ – limb (other sites)	49	325	696		

Imaging Studies by Duplex

Tips/Rationale

The use of duplex ultrasound in the evaluation of the pathologies of native arteries of the lower extremities has probably increased steadily over the years (although no report of the prevalence of this testing modality is available). If one considers advances in technology and patient safety, this increase can be easily justified. Ultrasound is a safer method of evaluation than angiography, magnetic resonance angiography (MRA), or computed tomography angiography (CTA) and probably yields similar accuracy, specificity, and sensitivity. However, just as with the other diagnostic imaging techniques mentioned previously and despite the use of Doppler (pulsed or color), duplex ultrasound of native arteries generates mostly anatomic information, meaning that the overall physiology of the limb cannot be inferred or truly appreciated by this modality of testing. Therefore, it is recommended that duplex ultrasound be considered an adjunct test to a comprehensive physiologic test to evaluate the functionality of the lower extremities (see algorithm). As such, duplex ultrasound can be easily tailored to specific areas of concern determined by physiologic testing, and the testing time (which is rather long for a full evaluation of both extremities) can be adapted and reduced depending on the information needed.

Duplex ultrasound, however, has significant use for follow-up of revascularization procedures and particularly bypass grafts (although an ankle-brachial index [ABI] should always be an integral part of the exam protocol because, again, it yields useful overall physiologic or functional information). Although the exam can be tedious (if the sonographer does not have access to the notes about the procedure), it has been proven to have great accuracy, sensitivity, and specificity.

The main question with any revascularization procedure is:

- Did the procedure achieve its goal? In other words, are the patient's symptoms relieved, has the patient regained function or gained more functions in his or her legs, and are there any side effects or remaining limitations?

Thus, the main areas to investigate are:

■ The inflow to the graft (or stent). Is it providing expected flow?

■ The proximal anastomoses of the graft (or proximal aspect of the stent). Is it allowing for flow to be diverted through the graft?

■ The main body of the graft (or stent). Is there any mechanical impairment to the flow (valve, kink, external compression, etc.) or any internal restriction of flow (thrombus, intimal hyperplasia, etc.)?

■ The distal anastomoses (or distal aspect of the stent). Is the diameter of the two conduits compatible? Is the stent placed correctly within the vessel lumen? Are there any other complications impeding the flow?

■ Finally, the outflow. Is there still significant disease distal to the revascularization site? Is most of the flow reaching the compromised tissue? Is the native system impaired (did the revascularization bypass collaterals)? These last questions, when the patient cannot really point to any improvement, may necessitate another full physiologic study to be compared with the preoperative exam.

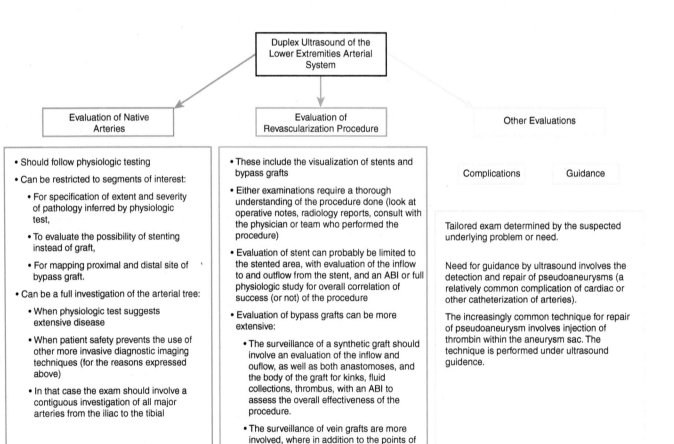

FIGURE 9.26.   Algorithm for examination.

Test Preparation

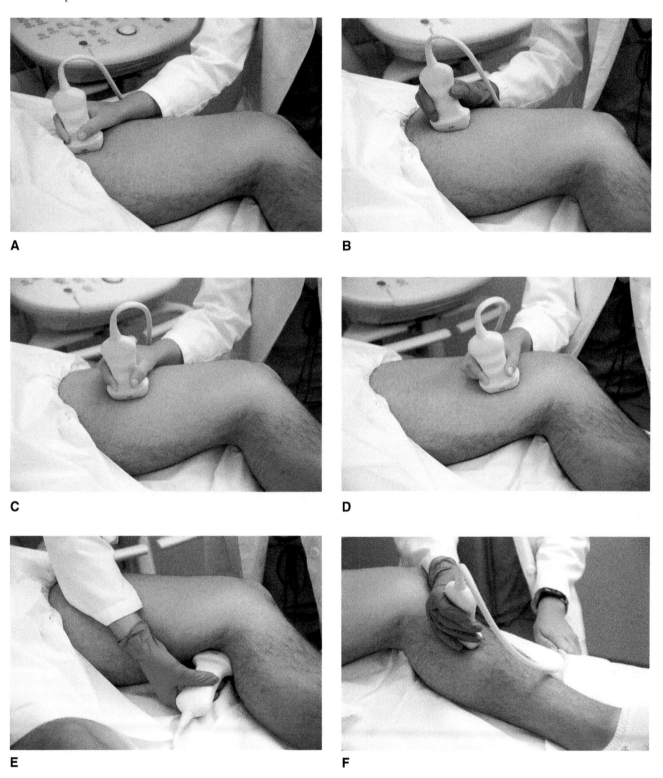

FIGURE 9.27. Evaluation sequence of the lower extremities arterial system in longitudinal view. (Continued)

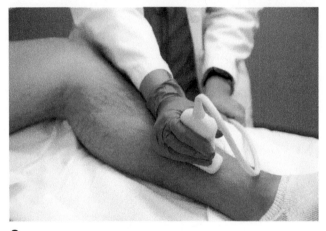

G

FIGURE 9.27. (Continued)

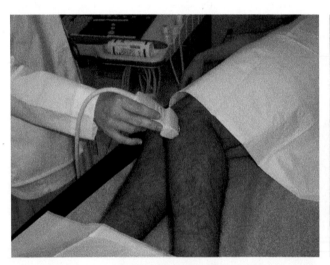

A

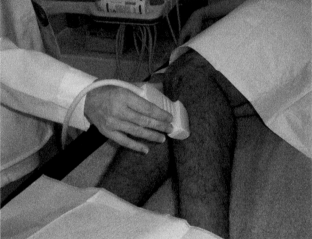

B

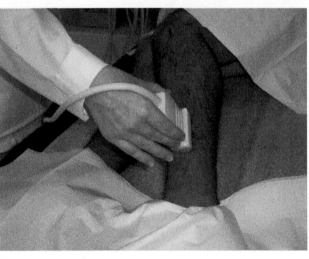

C

FIGURE 9.28.   Position required for the evaluation of the peroneal arteries or grafts that follow a lateral route (usually those with distal anastomoses at the anterior tibial artery).

Testing Sequence

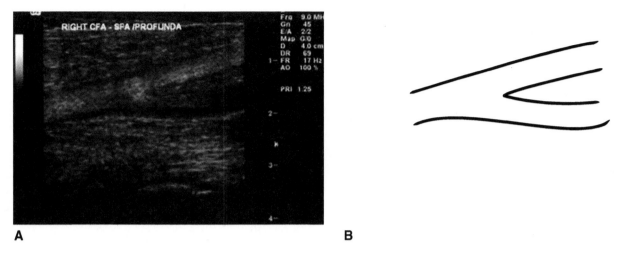

A   **B**

FIGURE 9.29.   Common femoral artery (CFA) and superficial femoral artery (SFA)/deep femoral artery (DFA) bifurcation with B flow. Full arterial duplex of the native arteries should start (at a minimum) at the CFA and proceed through the SFA/DFA bifurcation.

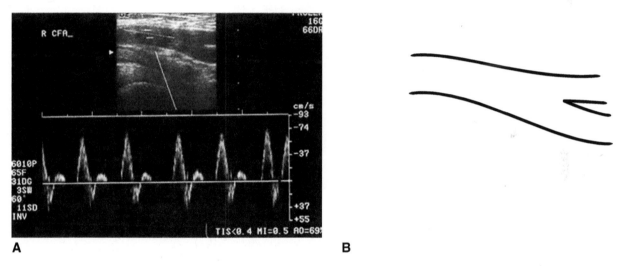

A   **B**

FIGURE 9.30.   Doppler (pulsed Doppler or pulsed wave) sample at the common femoral artery (CFA) with normal waveform and velocities.

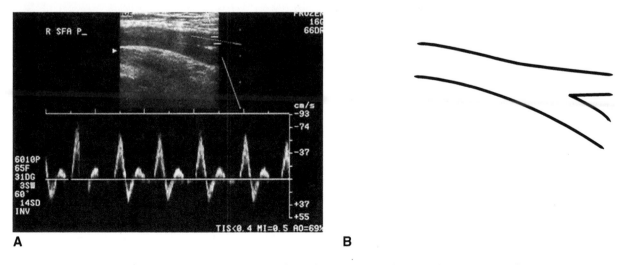

A   **B**

FIGURE 9.31.   Doppler sample at the proximal superficial femoral artery (SFA) with normal waveform and velocities.

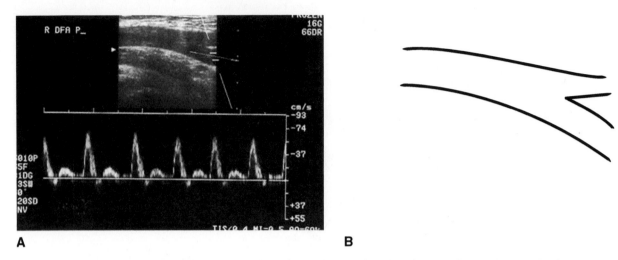

FIGURE 9.32.   Doppler sample at the proximal deep femoral artery (DFA) with normal waveform and velocities.

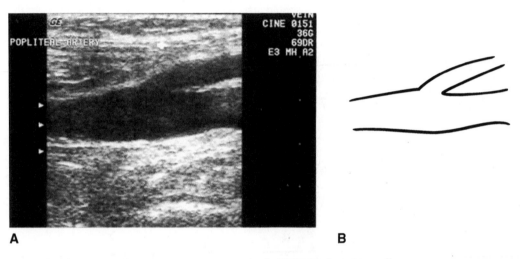

FIGURE 9.33.   Popliteal artery with gastrocnemius artery branching.

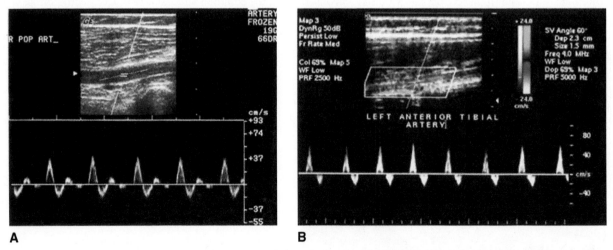

FIGURE 9.34.   Doppler samples at the popliteal artery (A) and anterior tibial artery (B) with normal waveforms and velocities.

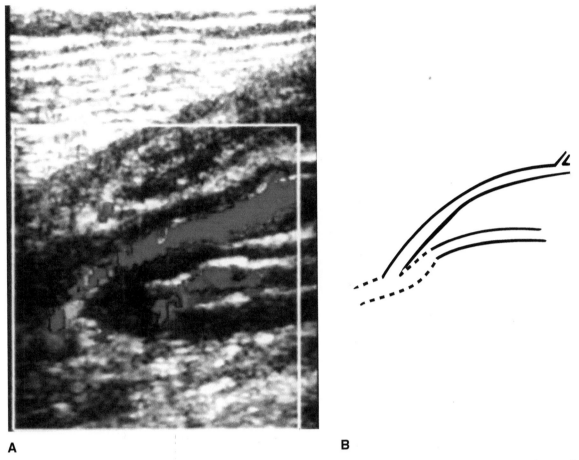

A   **B**

FIGURE 9.35.   Tibioperoneal trunk with bifurcation of the posterior tibial and peroneal arteries (the vessels not showing color fill are the paired posterior tibial and peroneal veins).

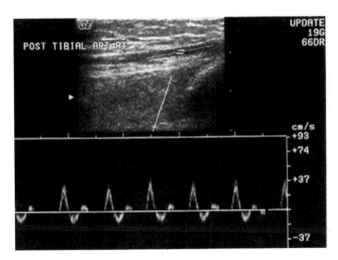

FIGURE 9.36.   Doppler sample at the posterior tibial artery with normal waveforms and velocities.

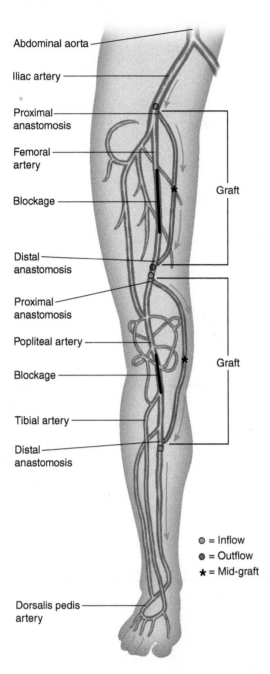

Abdominal aorta

Iliac artery

Proximal anastomosis

Femoral artery

Blockage

Distal anastomosis

Proximal anastomosis

Popliteal artery

Blockage

Tibial artery

Distal anastomosis

Graft

Graft

◐ = Inflow
● = Outflow
✱ = Mid-graft

Dorsalis pedis artery

FIGURE 9.37.   Points of special investigation for the evaluation of bypass grafts. The entire conduit should also be examined.

Results and Interpretation

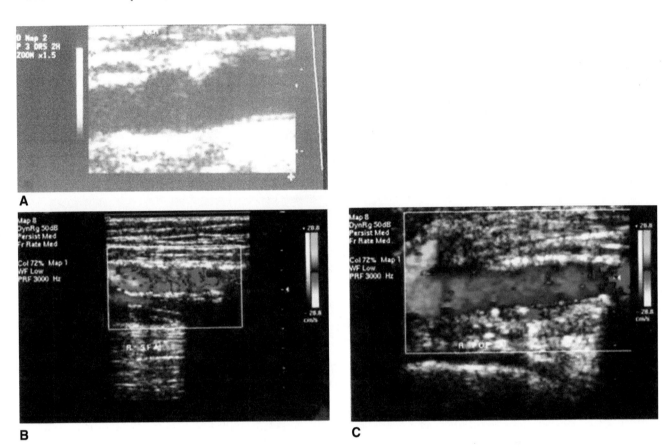

FIGURE 9.38. Diffuse atherosclerosis without significant flow restriction or stenosis. The intima appears thickened with areas of calcification.

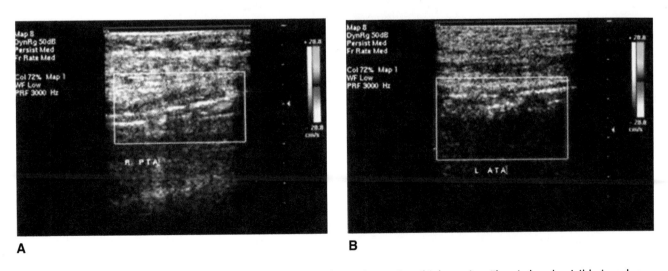

FIGURE 9.39. Calcification of small arteries, here a posterior and anterior tibial arteries. Flow is barely visible in color, although the arteries are not occluded. These vessels are probably noncompressible. The pathology resembles medial calcification or Mönckeberg's arteriosclerosis.

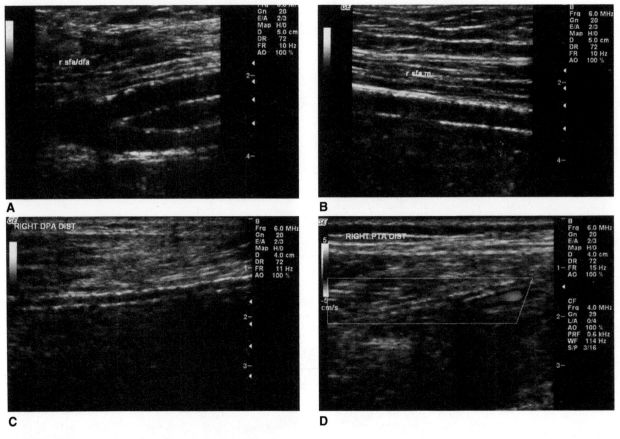

FIGURE 9.40. Examples of disseminated calcification of vessels without intimal plaque along the main arteries of the arterial tree of the lower extremities.

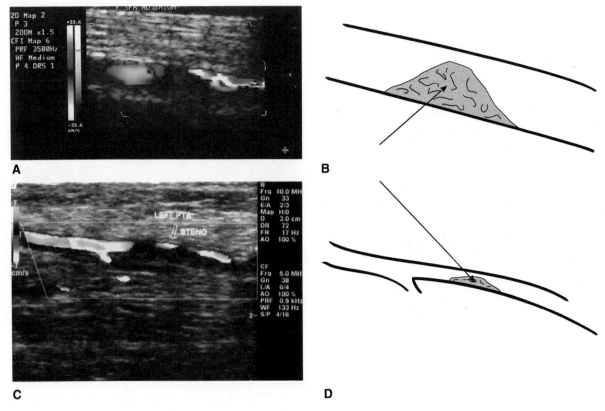

FIGURE 9.41. Soft plaque (arrows), homogenous and poorly echogenic and consistent with newly formed thrombus. The "mosaic" of colors distal to the stenosis suggests turbulence of flow and significant stenosis.

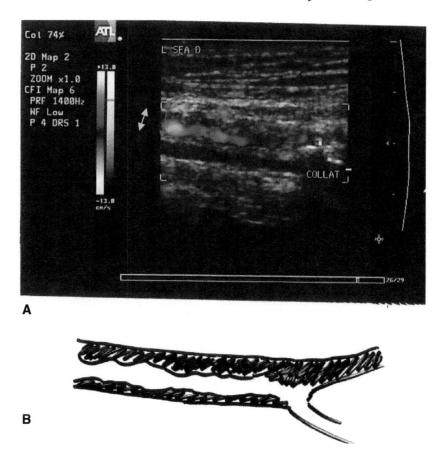

FIGURE 9.42. Significant atherosclerotic plaque along the vessel walls of this distal superficial femoral artery (the green double arrow represents the residual lumen, and the red double arrow represents the vessel's original diameter). An occlusion of the vessel is noted distal to the narrowing, as well as the presence of a collateral. This presentation will be seen in a long-standing, slow-developing disease process. Note: Revascularization by a bypass graft may compromise the collaterals.

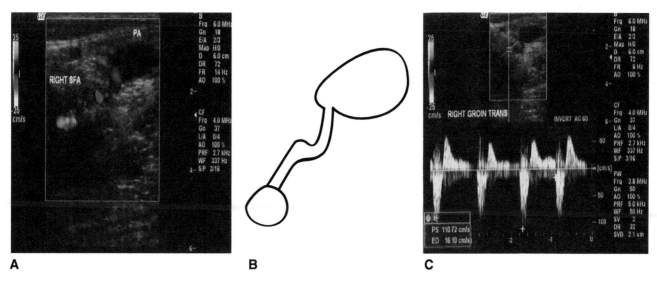

FIGURE 9.43. Pseudoaneurysm emerging from a superficial femoral artery (SFA) after cardiac catheterization. Visible "neck" (from needle track) can be seen linking the vessel and the pseudoaneurysm. Such a presentation may be feasible for compression and thrombin injection without too much risk of occluding the native vessel. Doppler waveforms (C) taken within the "neck" of the pseudoaneurysm display a typical pattern of flow to and fro (toward the aneurysm sac first and then reversed and toward the artery).

CHAPTER 9

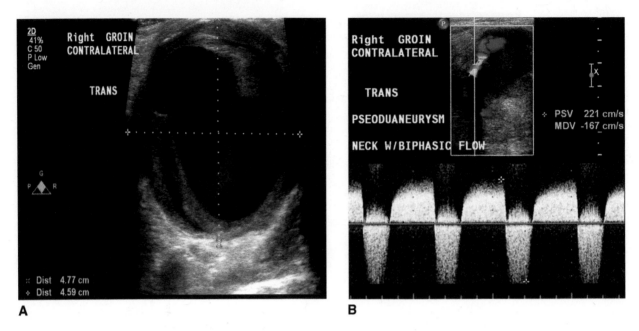

FIGURE 9.44. Pseudoaneurysm in a patient with a history of multiple vascular reconstruction in the left lower extremity. The right common femoral artery was used repeatedly as access for invasive imaging studies. (A) Pseudoaneurysm sac with partial thrombosis along the edge. However, the sac is large, and the flow (demonstrated in B) does not allow for spontaneous thrombosis. The well-delineated neck may allow for safe thrombosis of the pseudoaneurysm sac by thrombin injection. (B) Doppler waveforms taken within the "neck" of the pseudoaneurysm displaying a typical pattern of flow to and fro (toward the aneurysm sac first and then reversed and toward the artery).

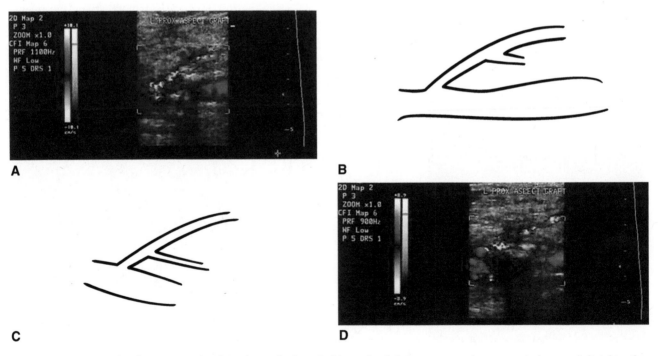

FIGURE 9.45. Proximal anastomosis of a vein graft. A untied branch of the greater saphenous vein is noted distal to the anastomosis, stealing flow from the graft.

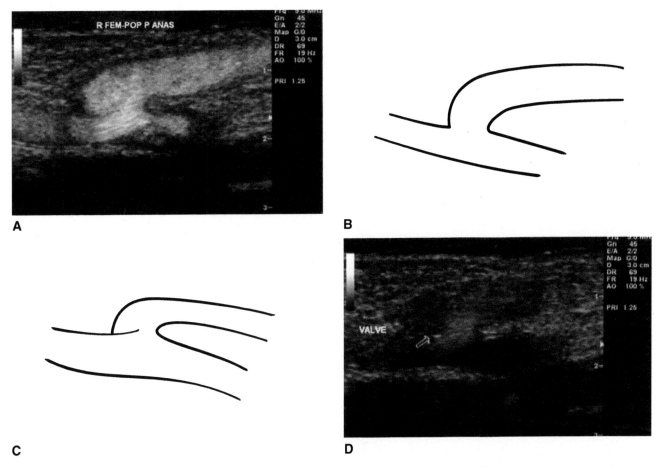

FIGURE 9.46. Proximal anastomosis of a vein graft, with B flow (A). The flow pattern suggests a "jet" of flow from the native common femoral artery (CFA) toward the graft. On further analysis, a retained valve is creating a stenosis with turbulent flow.

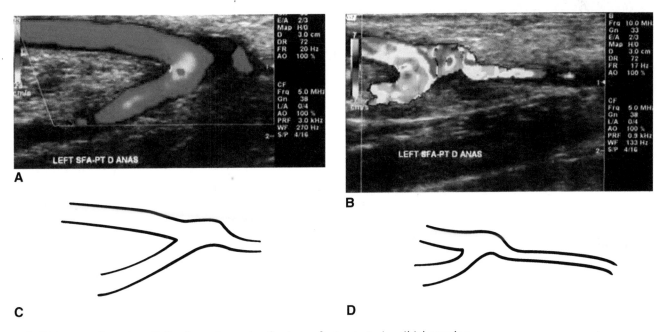

FIGURE 9.47. Samples of distal anastomosis of vein grafts to posterior tibial arteries.

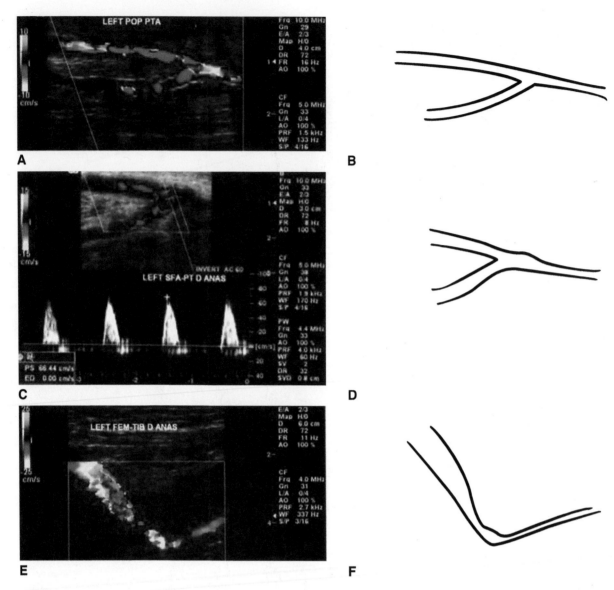

FIGURE 9.48. Sample of distal anastomosis of a vein graft to a much deeper tibial vessel, the peroneal artery.

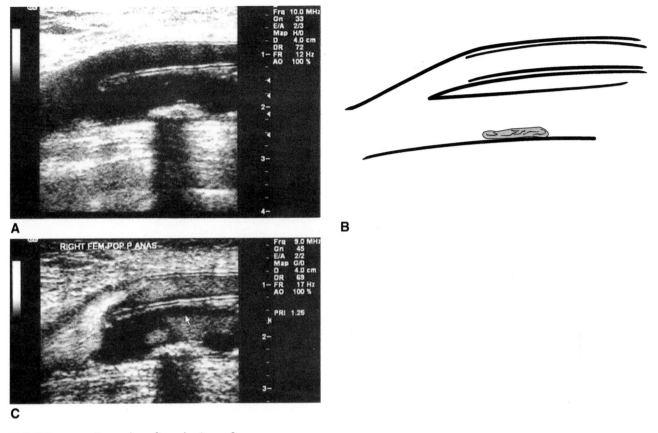

A

B

C

FIGURE 9.49.   Examples of synthetic grafts.

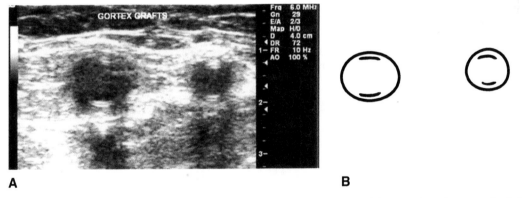

A

B

FIGURE 9.50.   Examples of multiple procedures. Two synthetic grafts are noted here. When these grafts fail, they are not typically removed (because they are often tunneled between fascia and muscles).

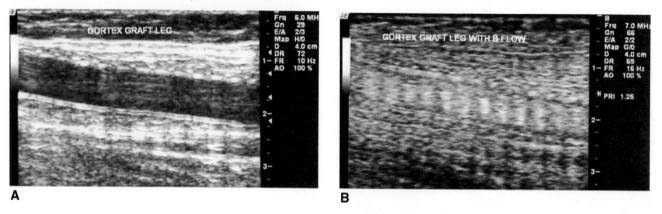

A   **B**

FIGURE 9.51.   Example of a typical appearance of a Gortex graft. The "ridges" of the graft material give an uneven appearance of flow on B flow.

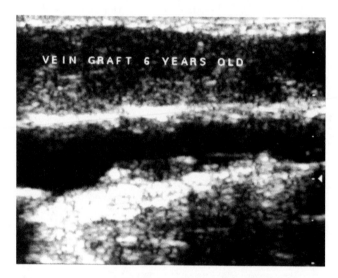

FIGURE 9.52.   Development of atherosclerotic plaque within a vein graft. Such pathology is not often observed but would lead to questions concerning the long-term patency of the graft.

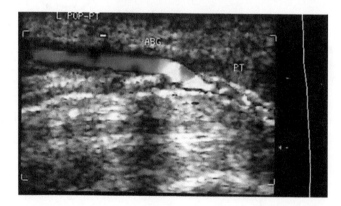

FIGURE 9.53.   There is presence of significant disease in the outflow vessel from this vein graft. The progression of disease in the outflow can greatly compromise the patency of the graft.

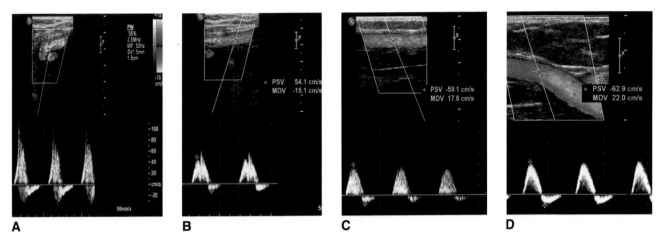

A   **B**   **C**   **D**

FIGURE 9.54.   Series of points of interest in graft surveillance, right common femoral to distal popliteal arterial bypass graft: series of color and pulse Doppler along a common femoral to distal popliteal arterial bypass vein graft. Both color and pulse Doppler spectrum and velocity measurements show no evidence of significant change of velocities or turbulence.

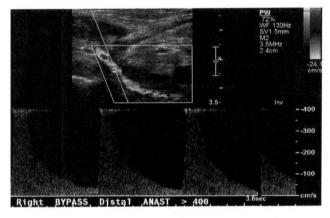

FIGURE 9.55.   Critical stenosis at the distal anastomosis of a right femoral to tibial artery bypass graft.

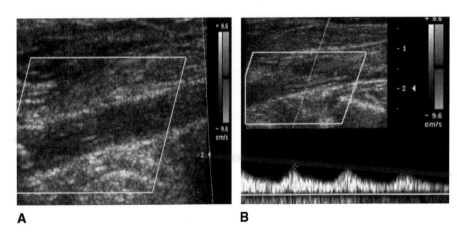

A   **B**

FIGURE 9.56.   Recanalization of an occluded artery (usually from collaterals) with very slow flow. Note that the color scale is set low. The velocity was recorded at 11 cm/s. The Doppler waveforms show delay in systole, rounded peak in systole, no temporary reverse flow in early diastole, or slight forward flow in late diastole.

TABLE 9.2 **Velocity Criteria for Interpretation of Stenosis or Occlusion within a Native Artery, Stent, or Bypass Graft Conduit**

What?	Normal	Mild, < 50% (determine point of highest velocity)	Moderate, > 50% (determine point of highest velocity)	Severe, > 75% (determine point of highest velocity)	Occlusion
How?	No evidence of plaque, flow restriction, turbulence with either color or pulsed Doppler	Focal increase of velocity from a proximal segment free of disease to a segment with some visible signs of disease; the velocity (peak systolic) in the diseased segment will be less than double that of the normal more proximal segment	Follow same approach as previous section; the velocity in the diseased segment will here be at least double that of the more proximal normal segment	Follow same approach as previous sections; the velocity in the diseased segment will be at least three times higher than that of the more proximal normal segment	No flow detected

The presence or absence of collaterals should be investigated and noted

Concluding Tips

Investigating the arterial circulation of the lower extremities is rather straightforward. The main tissues receiving flow are skeletal muscles directly involved in the functionality of the limbs, and their functions cannot be carried out efficiently without oxygen. As such, any decrease in the amount of oxygen and thus arterial flow delivered to the muscle or muscle groups will lead to symptoms when metabolic demand is increased and, ultimately, at rest. True symptoms of arterial insufficiency will be directly linked to the demand and supply, will be reproducible, and will lead to functional impairment. A comprehensive diagnosis should engender a tailored intervention and could ultimately be the most rewarding achievement in modern medicine because the patient could regain function of the tissue. I believe that the role of the vascular sonographer takes its full value in this area of testing.

CHAPTER
10

PART FOUR: PELVIS AND LOWER EXTREMITIES

Testing the Venous Circulation

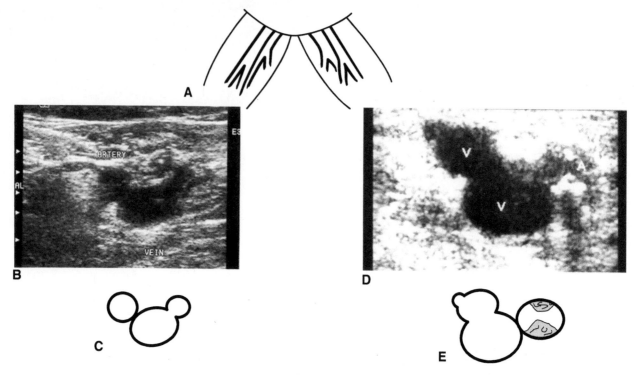

FIGURE 10.1.   Relative position of the common femoral artery and vein below the inguinal ligament. From lateral to medial, you should have: nerve, artery, vein, lymph nodes (NAVL on the right, lateral to medial, and LVAN on the left, medial to lateral).

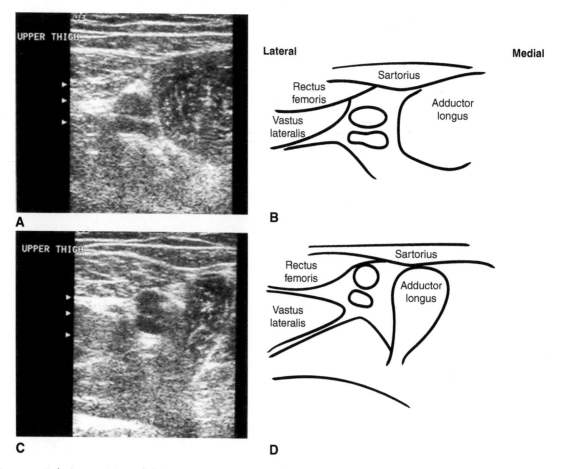

FIGURE 10.2.   Relative position of the major vessels (arteries and veins) and adjacent muscles in the lower extremities.

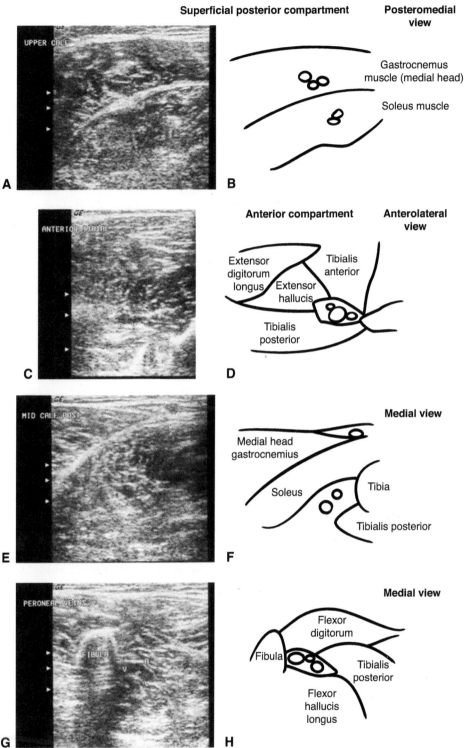

FIGURE 10.3.   Relative position of the major vessels (arteries and veins) and adjacent muscles in the lower extremities.

General Concepts in Venous Circulation

Tips/Rationale

If there is one area of diagnostic imaging where duplex ultrasound has found a primordial role for rapid, safe, and accurate diagnosis, it is in the evaluation of lower extremity venous circulation. Most other techniques, such as physiologic testing by air plethysmography (APG), impedance plethysmography (IPG), or even venography, have become obsolete. Although venograms are still performed, because of their invasive nature, they are usually reserved for special cases. Duplex ultrasound offers a safe and rapid evaluation of the major pathologic findings of the venous system (i.e., valvular incompetence and thrombosis) without the necessity of adding other diagnostic modalities for the initiation of treatment. Therefore, this chapter will only describe the imaging technique of lower extremity veins by duplex ultrasound, as well as the results and interpretation linked to symptoms pointing to either thrombosis or valvular incompetence.

The most important tips for a successful examination are:

- Keep in mind (always) that for venous diseases, and particularly deep vein thrombosis, there may not be clear clinical symptoms (unlike for arterial insufficiency).

- Remember to question the patient thoroughly about his/her history. Despite most popular beliefs, deep vein thrombosis (DVT) does not solely appear with a prolonged period of sitting or lying down. Indeed, patients recovering in hospital beds or rehabilitation centers or confined in nursing homes, although experiencing prolonged periods of immobilization, are also subjected to changes triggered by surgery, an underlying disease (cancer, errors of metabolism pathways, hypercoagulability, etc.), or other conditions, and these could be the triggering factors to the development of DVT for a more substantial portion of patients than the immobilization itself.

- Trauma, mechanical compression of more central veins, and rare neoplastic diseases of veins are also possible causes of DVT.

- On another note, several conditions not linked to venous problems can also induce similar clinical symptoms, such as Baker's cyst, muscle tears, hematoma, fistula, etc.

- The most important tip of all is to understand the limitations of the test. Although ultrasound is safe, easy to perform, and offers immediate and usually accurate results, it can only maintain these qualifications if the exam is performed thoroughly and all veins can be accessed. It is not unusual to have limited visualization, particularly in the pelvis, at the adductor's canal, and at the level of the tibial veins. A clear understanding of these limitations should prompt the sonographer to be cautious in his or her report to the physician, and areas of poor visualization should be noted as such (to report the remote yet real possibility that something was missed).

Protocol Algorithms

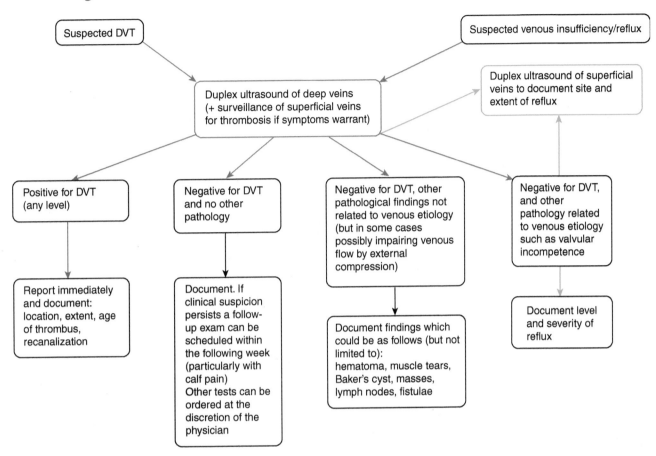

```
Suspected DVT ─────────────────┐                          ┌───────────── Suspected venous insufficiency/reflux

                    Duplex ultrasound of deep veins                Duplex ultrasound of superficial
                    (+ surveillance of superficial veins           veins to document site and
                    for thrombosis if symptoms warrant)            extent of reflux
```

| Positive for DVT (any level) | Negative for DVT and no other pathology | Negative for DVT, other pathological findings not related to venous etiology (but in some cases possibly impairing venous flow by external compression) | Negative for DVT, and other pathology related to venous etiology such as valvular incompetence |

| Report immediately and document: location, extent, age of thrombus, recanalization | Document. If clinical suspicion persists a follow-up exam can be scheduled within the following week (particularly with calf pain) Other tests can be ordered at the discretion of the physician | Document findings which could be as follows (but not limited to): hematoma, muscle tears, Baker's cyst, masses, lymph nodes, fistulae | Document level and severity of reflux |

FIGURE 10.4. Algorithm for examination.

Imaging Studies by Duplex

Test Preparation

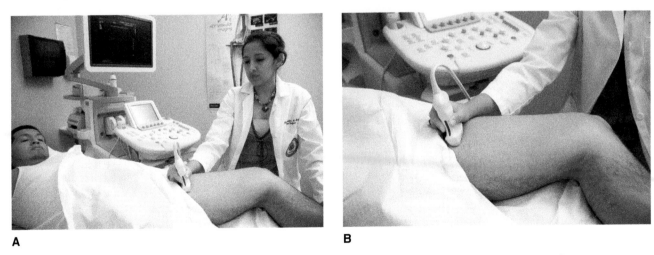

A

B

FIGURE 10.5. Patient position and exam sequence for assessing vein compressibility to rule out DVT. The exam starts with the transducer placed in transverse position below the inguinal ligament (A). (Continued)

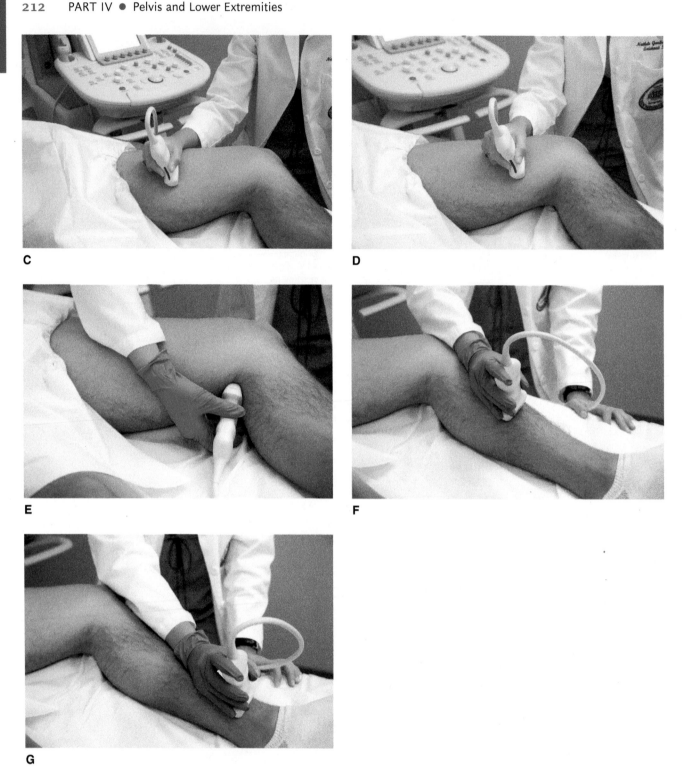

FIGURE 10.5.   The exam continues by performing compression of the veins at all levels (making sure complete compression of the vessel can be achieved before moving to the next segment). The transducer should be moved one transducer width at a time so the entire length of the vessel is visualized and examined (A through G). At the level of the popliteal fossa (E) the transducer can be moved first slightly proximally to examine the vessels at the adductor canal (aka Hunter's canal), then distally to examine the upper calf vessels, which include the distal popliteal vein, the tibioperoneal trunk, but also the gastrocnemius muscle veins. The transducer will then be placed in the medial aspect of the leg to examine tibial paired veins—the posterior tibial and peroneal veins, as well as the soleal veins. The anterior tibial veins are usually not examined routinely due to low incidence of thrombosis. The superficial veins, the greater and lesser saphenous veins, can be examined at the same time (medial approach for greater saphenous vein and posterior approach from the popliteal fossa for the lesser saphenous vein).

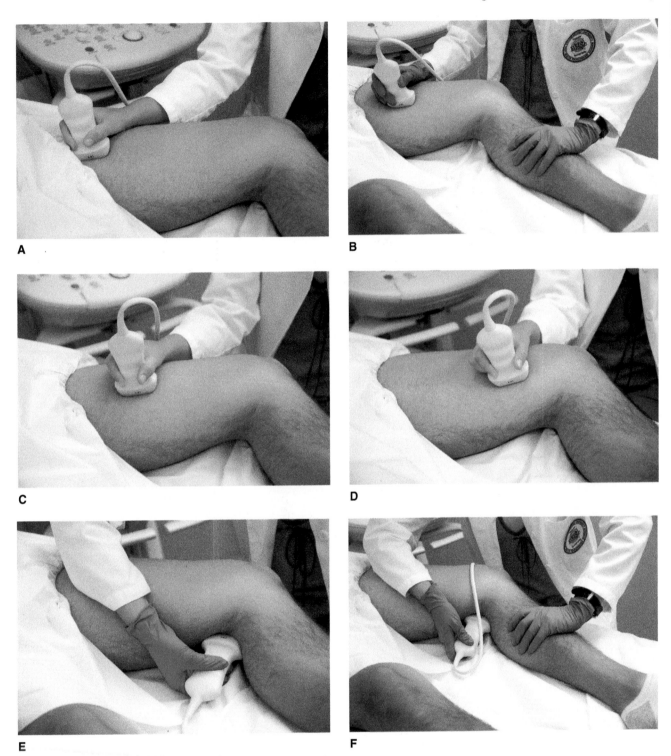

FIGURE 10.6. Patient position and exam sequence for performing Doppler assessment for valve competence and flow characteristics. The transducer is placed in a longitudinal position and the exam starts at the level of the inguinal ligament to assess flow in the common femoral vein (A). Note that the sonographer also squeezes the calf intermittently. This maneuver should be performed with the image displaying either color Doppler or PW Doppler so valve competence could be assessed. The transducer will be moved one transducer length at a time, so all veins should be assessed (A through H). (Continued)

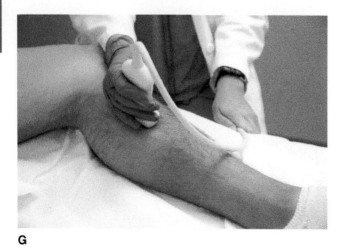

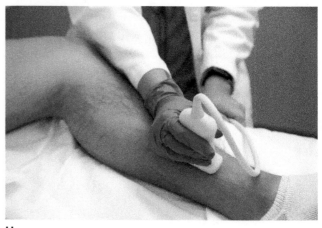

G   **H**

FIGURE 10.6.   (Continued)

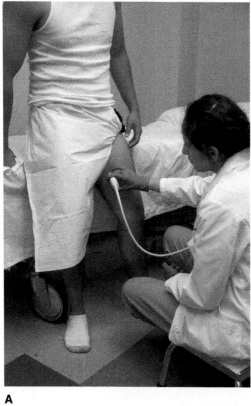

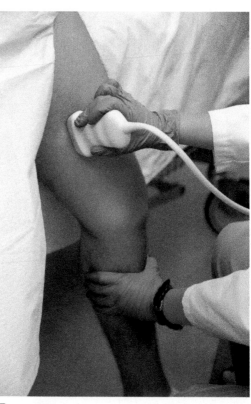

A   **B**

FIGURE 10.7.   Preferred position for evaluation of valvular incompetence prior to vein ablation. Caution: Many patients will not be able to remain in this position. The sonographer should also make sure that his or her position is comfortable.

Testing Sequence

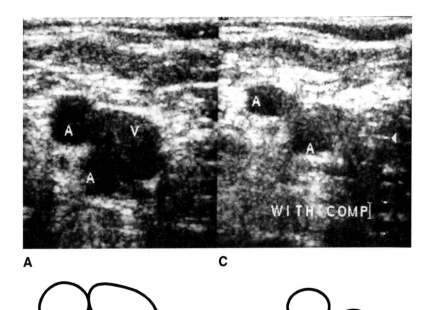

FIGURE 10.8. Normal compression in gray scale at the level of the common femoral vein. Split image shows complete compression of the common femoral vein, thus excluding DVT.

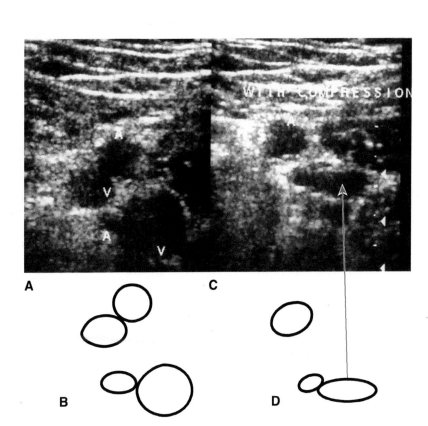

FIGURE 10.9. Normal compression in gray scale at the level of the superficial femoral/deep femoral veins. Split image shows complete compression of the femoral vein (i.e., superficial femoral vein) but incomplete compression of the deep femoral vein (see arrow). In this case, another approach or technique, such as color Doppler or power Doppler, should be used to ensure and document patency of that vein.

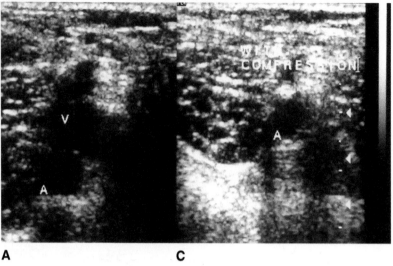

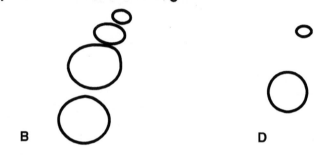

FIGURE 10.10. Normal compression in gray scale of the popliteal vein. Split images show full compression of all veins displayed and evaluated. Evaluation of these veins is best done through a posterior approach.

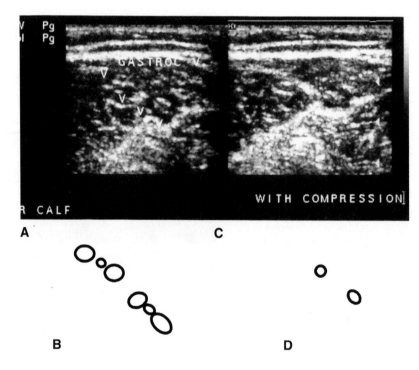

FIGURE 10.11. Normal compression in gray scale of the gastrocnemius muscle veins. Split images show full compression of all veins displayed and evaluated. Evaluation of these veins is best done through a posterior approach. The gastrocnemius veins should always be examined, and particular attention should be paid to these veins if the patient complains of calf pain. These are prone to thrombosis from prolonged immobilization independent of underlying disease.

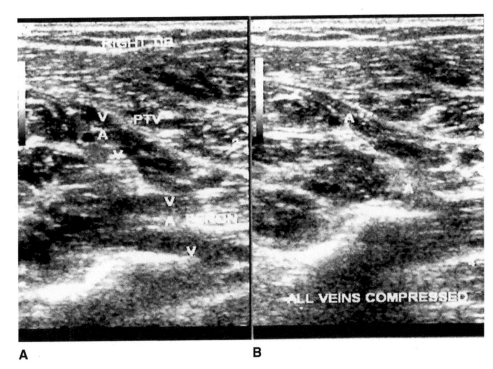

FIGURE 10.12. Normal compression in gray scale of the posterior tibial and peroneal veins. Split images show full compression of all veins displayed and evaluated. Evaluation of these veins is usually done through a medial approach. Note: The anterior tibial veins are usually not evaluated unless thrombosis is suspected. These veins have only rarely been documented as prone to thrombosis, independent of the underlying cause for hypercoagulability. However, all posterior tibial and peroneal veins should be included. The soleal veins can also be included if symptoms correlate and no other pathology has been noted.

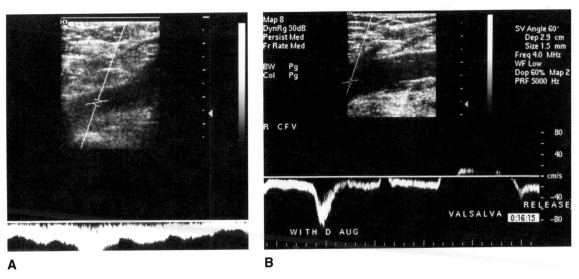

FIGURE 10.13. Normal pulse Doppler at the common femoral vein. The deep veins should be interrogated by Doppler and/or color. Normal venous hemodynamic should show spontaneous flow, phasicity with respiration, and response to maneuvers. Caution: These do not make the duplex exam a physiologic study. (A) Shows: Spontaneous signal (without maneuvers, flow is detectable) and phasicity with respiration (the signal undulates slightly with each breath cycle). (B) Shows: Normal response to distal augmentation (when the lower thigh or calf is "squeezed," flow is forcefully sent through the vein more proximally) and normal response to Valsalva maneuver (flow stops during forceful inhalation, and then resumes with exhalation).

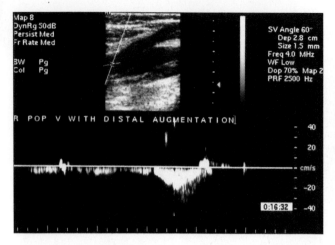

FIGURE 10.14. Normal pulse Doppler at the popliteal vein. Note: The entire venous system does not need to be interrogated by Doppler. A minimum documentation should include the common femoral vein, the popliteal vein, and the tibial veins. Shows: Spontaneity of signal, phasicity of signal, and normal response to distal augmentation.

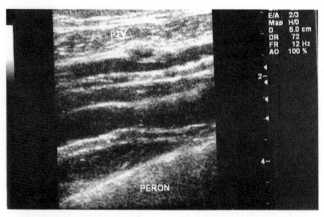

FIGURE 10.15. Enlarged veins could be suspicious for acute DVT. Compression would have to ensure that no DVT was present. Pulse Doppler is sometimes difficult to perform in these veins; therefore, color Doppler is preferably used to demonstrate complete filling of the veins as seen in Figure 10.16.

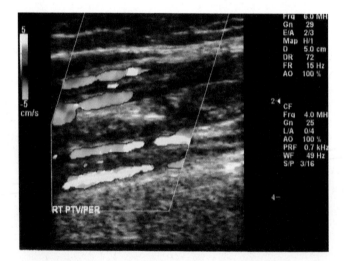

FIGURE 10.16. Normal color Doppler tibial veins. Demonstration of patency of posterior tibial and peroneal veins with color Doppler. Note: The color scale is set rather low. The flow in tibial veins is often slow and sluggish. In real-time scanning, the color should be left on while performing distal augmentation maneuvers to demonstrate a rise in flow, as seen previously on the Doppler spectrum.

Results and Interpretation

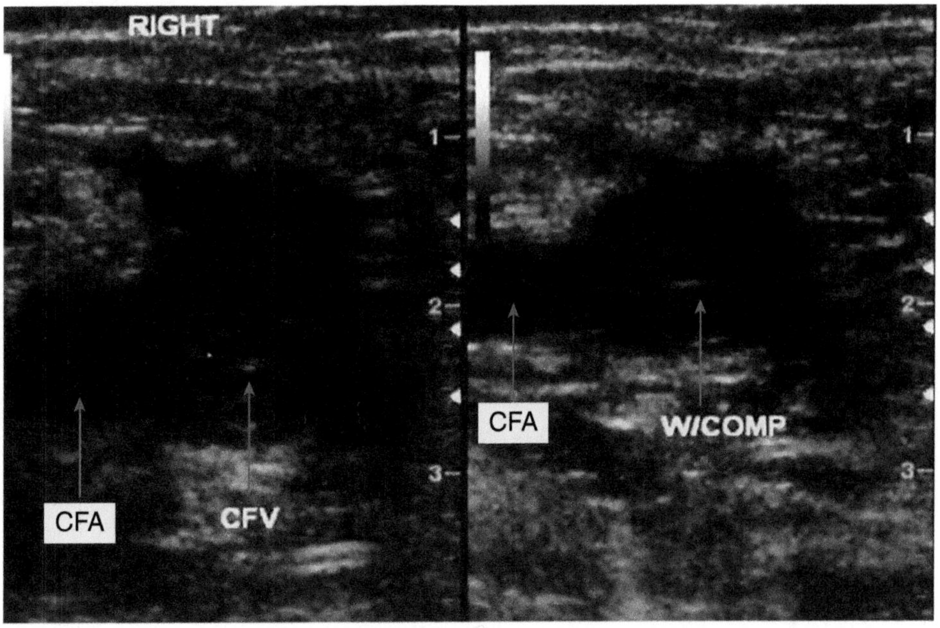

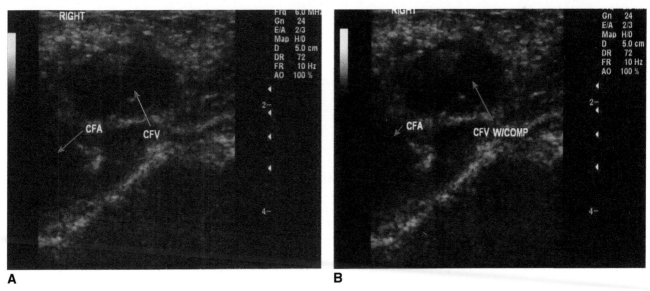

FIGURE 10.17. Acute thrombosis of the common femoral vein. The vein is significantly distended compared to the artery, and the lumen is filled with anechoic material. This suggests acute thrombosis (pulsed and/or color Doppler would allow one to determine if the thrombus is occluding the vessel or not).

FIGURE 10.18. Slightly organized thrombus of the common femoral vein. Compression of this common femoral vein shows no compression. The vein is not overdistended compared to the artery, and echogenic material is seen within the vein lumen. This usually suggests that the process is several days old, with the thrombus starting to become organized with fibrin deposit.

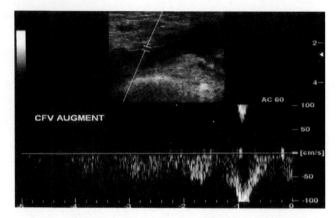

FIGURE 10.19. Abnormal pulse Doppler in common femoral vein. This Doppler spectrum was taken with the slightly organized thrombus shown in Figure 10.18. The Doppler spectrum shows slight loss of phasicity of the signal and higher flow velocity, which may suggest some proximal extension although not occlusion. The normal distal augmentation suggests that there is probably no significant distal extension of the thrombus.

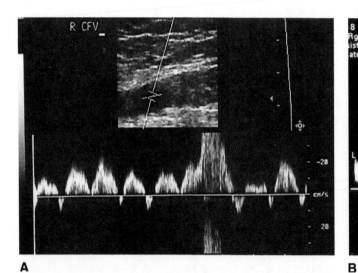

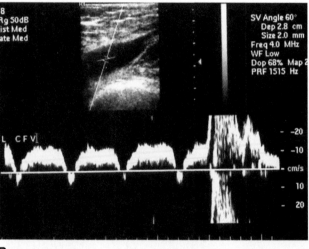

A   **B**

FIGURE 10.20. Abnormal pulse Doppler in common femoral vein. Pulsatile flow is demonstrated in the right and left common femoral veins. This finding is often bilateral and can be seen occasionally in well-hydrated and physically active young individuals. It is most often seen in patients with increased central pressure, such as with right-sided congestive heart failure. The increased central pressure contributes to the pulsatility pattern due to transmission of cardiac pulsation.

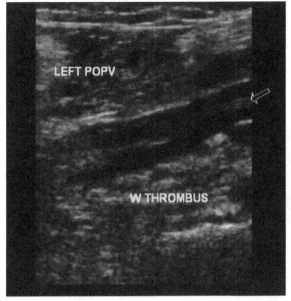
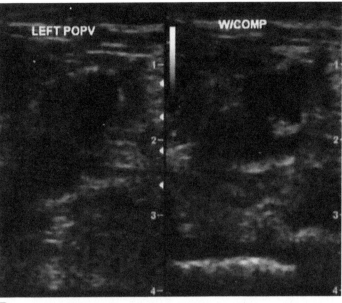

A   **B**

FIGURE 10.21.   Subacute thrombosis in the popliteal vein: popliteal vein with thrombus in longitudinal and transverse views. The thrombus appears more echogenic in longitudinal view, and the vein is not significantly distended. This may suggest subacute thrombosis. Note: There is really no significant importance to note the relative "age" of the thrombus, except for follow-up and in newly referred patients who are already being treated for thrombosis (although these considerations are important for the treating physician).

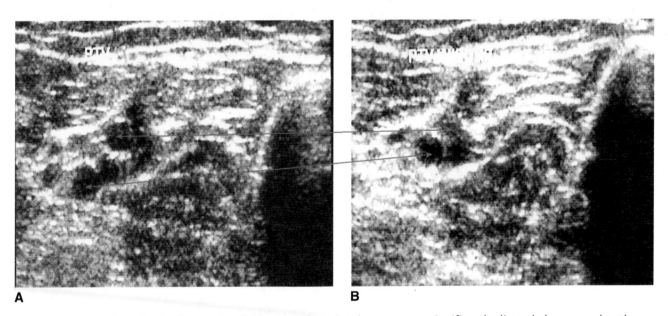

A   **B**

FIGURE 10.22.   Thrombosis of posterior tibial veins. The veins do not appear significantly distended compared to the artery. However, the veins are not compressible, and the thrombus material is not echogenic. These findings point to probable acute thrombosis, despite the lack of distension. However, because tibial veins are usually small, they do not tend to distend too dramatically, even with acute thrombosis compared to a larger vein, such as the common femoral or popliteal vein.

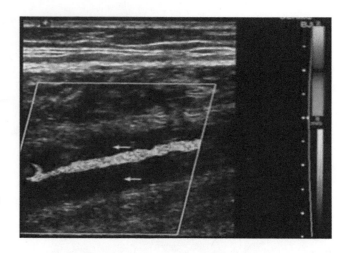

FIGURE 10.23. Thrombosis of the paired tibial veins diagnosed with color Doppler. The posterior tibial artery displays flow with color Doppler, but despite distal augmentation, color is not seen in either of the paired veins. The veins also appear slightly distended, and the thrombus material is only slightly echogenic, suggesting an acute to subacute process.

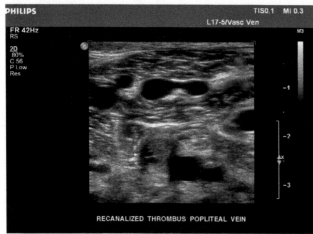

A

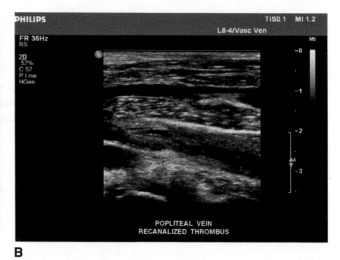

B

FIGURE 10.24. Recanalized thrombus in popliteal veins. Even on this gray scale images a portion of the lumen is visible without echogenic material. Caution: Color Doppler should be used to ensure recanalization (versus superimposed acute thrombotic process) as in Figure 10.25. Courtesy of Philips.

FIGURE 10.25. Recanalized thrombus in femoral vein with color. Courtesy of Philips.

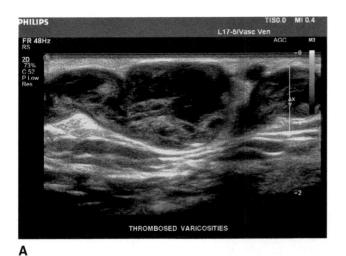

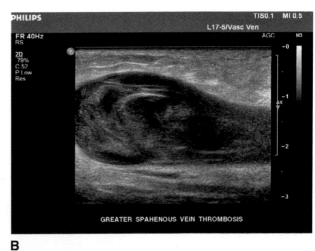

A   B

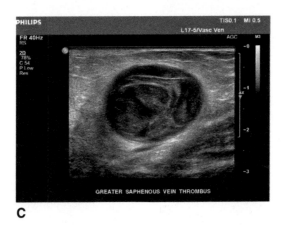

C

FIGURE 10.26. Varicosities with thrombus in greater saphenous vein. Courtesy of Philips.

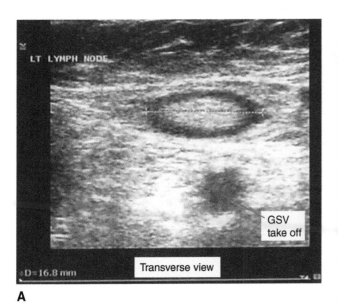

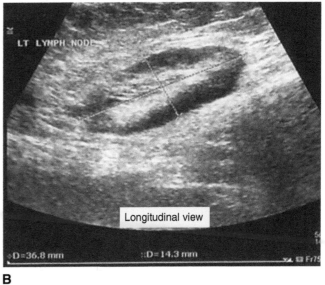

A   B

FIGURE 10.27. Enlarged lymph nodes in the left inguinal area. These should be evaluated in both longitudinal and transverse views to ensure that they are not mistaken for thrombosis in veins, such as the greater saphenous vein or a branch of that system. Indeed, lymph nodes are anatomically located medially and close to veins.

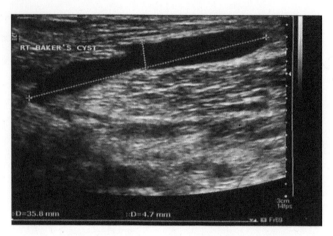

FIGURE 10.28. Baker's cyst in popliteal fossa. Baker's cysts result from inflammation of the synovial sac with accumulation of serous fluid. Because the popliteal fossa is a small space, the enlargement of the cyst by fluid accumulation may compress artery, vein, and nerve and cause discomfort, which may mimic DVT. In addition, because of heat, the inflammatory process may also mimic symptoms of DVT. Finally, Baker's cysts can rupture and cause pain in the upper calf area.

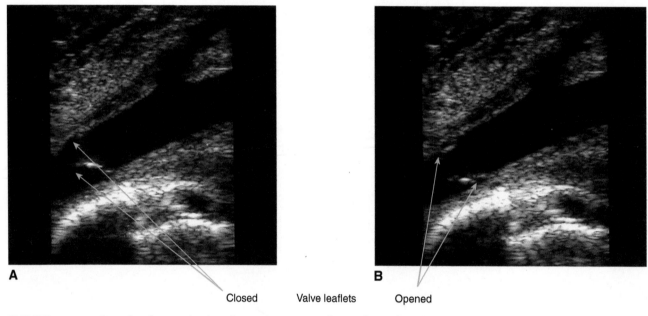

A   B

Closed   Valve leaflets   Opened

FIGURE 10.29. Sample of normal valve closure in common femoral vein (CFV).

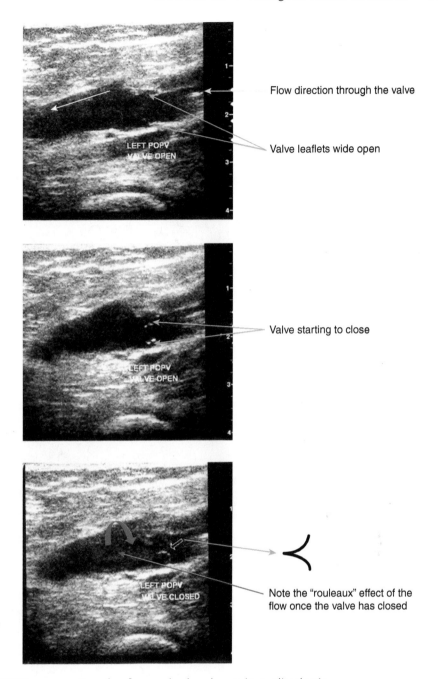

FIGURE 10.30.   Sample of normal valve closure in popliteal vein.

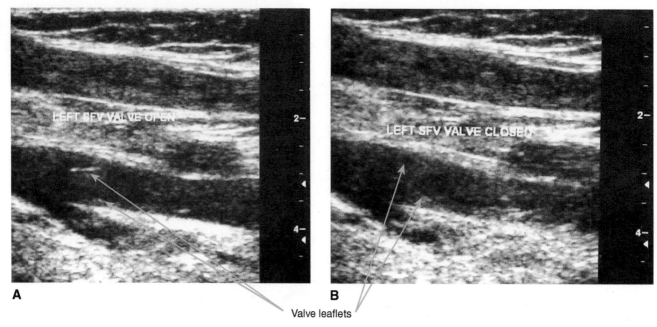

Valve leaflets

FIGURE 10.31.   Sample of normal valve closure in the superficial femoral vein (SFV).

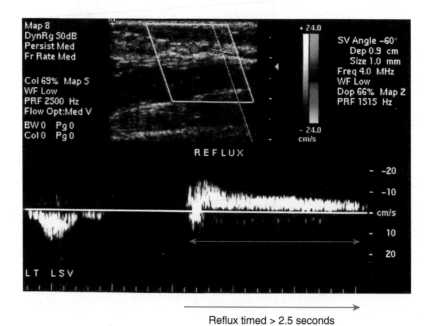

Reflux timed > 2.5 seconds

FIGURE 10.32.   Reflux by color Doppler and spectrum in the lesser saphenous vein (LSV).

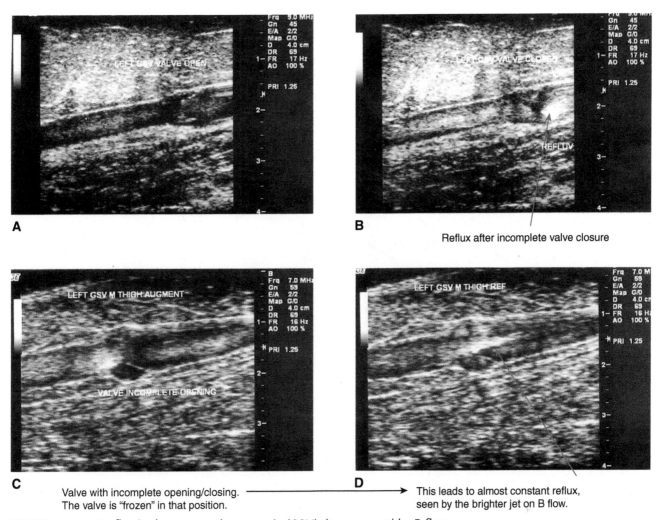

Reflux after incomplete valve closure

Valve with incomplete opening/closing. The valve is "frozen" in that position.

This leads to almost constant reflux, seen by the brighter jet on B flow.

FIGURE 10.33.   Reflux in the great saphenous vein (GSV) demonstrated by B flow.

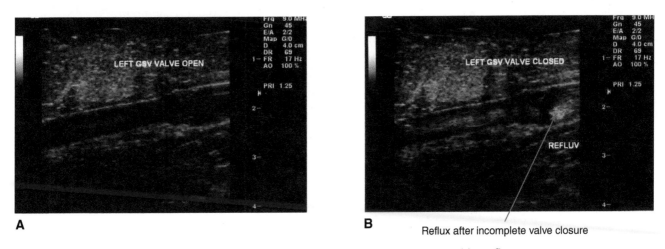

Reflux after incomplete valve closure

FIGURE 10.34.   Other sample of reflux in great saphenous vein (GSV) demonstrated by B flow.

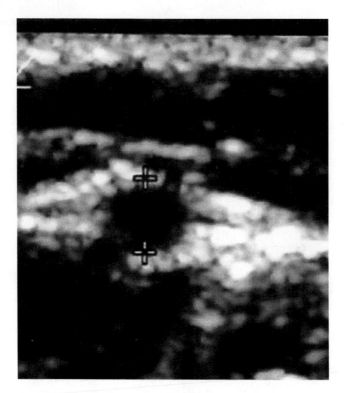

FIGURE 10.35. Measuring superficial vein (for subsequent use for bypass graft or for documentation of size before venous ablation). Note: The vein is measured preferably in anteroposterior dimension to ensure that the sonographer is not compressing the vessel and therefore is obtaining a true diameter. One ensures that the vein is not being compressed by looking at its shape (a rounder shape almost excludes compression).

TABLE 10.1: Valve Distribution on the Lower Extremities

Lower Extremity Vein	Valve Distribution	Normal Valvular Function
Iliac veins	None to one valve (25% of people)	Not reported
Common femoral vein	None to one valve (usually proximal to the saphenofemoral junction, at the level of the inguinal ligament)	Up to 1.5 seconds with Valsalva maneuver
Superficial femoral vein	One to four valves (typically three)	Up to 0.5 second reflux at valve closure
Popliteal vein	One to three valves (typically one)	Up to 0.5 second reflux at valve closure
Tibial veins	Approximately every inch	Up to 0.5 second reflux at valve closure
Superficial veins (greater and lesser saphenous)	Seven to nine valves (one valve is located at the saphenofemoral junction)	Up to 0.5 second reflux at valve closure
Perforator veins	One to two valves	Up to 0.5 second reflux at valve closure
Soleal sinuses	No valves	N/A

Concluding Tips

The usefulness of duplex ultrasound as the sole test for the diagnosis of venous pathologies (i.e., thrombosis and valvular incompetence) has been well demonstrated. The greatest words of caution I would give would be as follows:

- Understand the limitations of correlation of clinical symptoms to test results.
- Always remain vigilant and thorough during an examination, particularly in demonstrating full compression of the vessels throughout the *entire length* (not just selected segments) of the vessels. The initial thrombosis can be very focal.
- Caution: The number of tests performed in a busy laboratory may trigger overconfidence! Performing a test in the vascular lab is not a race, even with large volume and understaffing, so take your time! With DVT, you cannot afford to miss anything.
- Always include tibial vessels and major calf veins in a full exam because pulmonary embolism can also arise from calf vein thrombosis.
- Document incidental findings. Cellulitis symptoms can mimic DVT, and enlarged lymph nodes would probably be present. Muscle tears or hematomas can trigger acute pain, so check the area of symptoms. Extrinsic compression (from masses) at the level of the pelvis can generate edema mimicking DVT. Newly enlarged superficial veins may indirectly point to deep venous problems.
- The positioning of patients for reflux study is still a matter of debate in some circles. My best recommendation is to always make sure the patient is comfortable throughout the test and that the sonographer does not expose himself or herself to musculoskeletal injury from an uncomfortable position. With that said:
  - Having the patient supine on the exam table and the table in reverse Trendelenburg position is acceptable. If symptoms are being caused by reflux, this will be demonstrated in that position just as well as it would be with the patient standing.
  - Many physicians are now being trained or have the opportunity to be trained by specialized seminars on assessing reflux. They should be familiar with visualization and additional mapping for performing venous ablation. However, I believe that this is beyond the scope of the sonographer's practice at this point.
- The sonographer's scope of practice in mapping venous reflux is to:
  - Clearly mark the proximal point of reflux.
  - Ensure that reflux is not caused by tributaries or problems with the deep venous system.
  - Ensure that the deep venous system is free of thrombus.
  - Ensure that the superficial veins are not major collaterals for occluded or ligated deep veins.

The Vascular Laboratory Beyond Techniques

PART I: Billing Essentials

Definitions

CPT Codes: Current Procedural Terminology (CPT). CPT codes are a set of codes, descriptions, and guidelines intended to describe procedures and services performed by physicians and other health care providers. CPT codes are revised every year, and the changes become effective as of January. Additionally, it is important that you become familiar with the definition of each CPT code used in vascular ultrasound. Each code represents a "billing" entity, and although some diseases/pathologies may warrant the use of several tests (even in the vascular laboratory), the sequence and choice of tests is also linked in our health care system to medical necessity and appropriate documentation from a referring physician. For example, even though performing a duplex scan to evaluate the specific location of a disease in the lower extremity arterial tree seems to be a logical second test to perform after a physiologic study does not mean that an insurance company or Medicare will look at it from that perspective! A well-developed algorithm with appropriate documentation is your best safeguard during a potential audit and also to ensure quality of care.

Modifiers: Modifiers are usually number or number/letter identifiers also described by the American Medical Association (AMA) in the CPT code book that allow for the modification of a code. In vascular laboratories for example, the code 93970 is used for complete duplex exam of the venous system and is the same code whether the test is performed for the lower or upper extremities. Most insurance companies would question using the same code twice on the same day. Using the modifier 59, for example, when billing for both duplex studies (i.e., for lower and upper extremities on the same day and same visit) would let insurance companies and/or Medicare know that you did the tests in two different sets of limbs, providing appropriate documentation to warrant doing both tests.

Code Bundle: Many procedures are now done in the same manner and follow a particular sequence of tasks or other "sub" procedures. To make the billing process easier to handle in these cases, the AMA put together special CPT codes that include all of these "sub" procedures so they do not have to be billed individually. For example, the codes for venous ablation by radiofrequency or laser of one or multiple veins for venous incompetence are 36475, 36476, 36478, and 36479. All of these codes are "bundles" of other codes, meaning that, for our purpose for example, they already include vein mapping by duplex prior to the procedure. Therefore, a 93970 or 93971 cannot be billed in addition immediately prior to the venous ablation (meaning, for the most part, on the same day).

Global Service: Some procedures or other services require a certain amount of time (in days, weeks, or months) before they can be billed for consecutively (unless special circumstances require the procedure, and usually, proof of need is required). For example, we just learned that 36475 and 93970 cannot be billed on the same day because the latter is part of the former. However, can they be billed on two different days? In fact, 36475 has a zero day global, meaning that a second procedure (if medically necessary) could be billed on the next consecutive day, or 93970 can be billed for the next day, if another evaluation is warranted.

ICD-9m Codes: International Classification of Disease, 9th Edition (ICD-9). This classification was started in 1955 by the World Health Organization (WHO) to serve as a means and classification method to study diseases and mortality causes with statistical analysis. It was subsequently modified for clinical purposes by the American Hospital Association (AHA) (*m* in ICD-9m stands for clinical modification from the WHO version). All diseases have been assigned a code. These codes are used for diagnosis purposes, and although different from the CPT codes, they are usually linked in that CPT codes will be deemed billable (in terms of being reimbursed by insurance) only for some specific ICD-9 codes. For example, a duplex scan of the extracranial arteries (CPT: 93880) can be justified for cerebral arterial disease (ICD-9: 437.9) but may raise questions for peripheral vascular disease (ICD-9: 443.9) and will certainly not get paid for gangrenous ulcer (ICD-9: 785.4). However, *never* tailor the ICD-9 code to the CPT code (unless you want to get audited for fraud)!

DRG: Diagnosis-Related Group (DRG). In 1980 during a study of clinical outcomes in hospitals, some 18,000 medical and 5,000 surgical ICD-9 codes were combined to create approximately 700 DRGs. Again, the idea was to "bundle" diagnostic tests, procedures, and treatment protocols under one payment schedule, with the rationale that each of these 700 or so DRGs represented a specific "admission" entity linked to the same type of test, treatment, or procedure, so independent of the patient, they should be paid with the same fee schedule. Basically the hospital receives a set lump sum for each of the DRGs, and anything done above and beyond the code is basically not paid for!

CPT Code Description, Use, and Restriction of Use

Note: When types of testing are listed in parenthesis, they are meant to be descriptions of the tests included in a specific category; this absolutely does not imply that *all* of the tests listed should be performed. The types of tests and the area investigated are determined by each laboratory and recorded on their written protocol. Basically the main part of the code definition to be concerned about is if the study is complete (bilateral) or limited (unilateral) and which limbs should be investigated (upper or lower extremity).

CPT Codes	Official Description	Appropriate Use and Restrictions
Cerebrovascular		
93875	Noninvasive physiologic studies of extracranial arteries, complete bilateral study (periorbital flow direction with arterial compression, ocular pneumoplethysmography, Doppler ultrasound spectral analysis)	Not used any longer (except for some research protocols)
93880	Duplex scan of extracranial arteries, <u>complete bilateral study</u>	Most often used today and usually includes scan of the extracranial carotid (CCA, ICA, and ECA at different levels) and vertebral arteries
93882	Duplex scan of extracranial arteries, <u>unilateral or limited study</u>	Would be used if only one side is scanned such as after a stent or endarterectomy or if, for some reason, only a portion of the protocol was followed
93886	Transcranial Doppler study of the intracranial arteries, <u>complete study</u>	Would be used usually for bilateral evaluation of the distal ICA, siphon, MAC, ACA, PCA, and basilar artery, but by Doppler or duplex, to check for vasospasm, reverse flow, stenosis, and occlusion
93888	Transcranial Doppler study of the intracranial artery, <u>limited study</u>	Would be used to evaluate specific arteries or just one side, usually after completion of procedure such as aneurysm clipping, etc.
Extremities Arterial		
93922	Noninvasive physiologic studies of the upper or lower extremity arteries, <u>single level</u>, bilateral (ankle/brachial index, Doppler waveform analysis, volume plethysmography, $TcPO_2$)	Cannot be billed alone without proof of waveforms (PVR, PPG, or CW) at that level; ABIs by themselves are normally part of the physical exam performed by the physician (and are bundled with the office visit); TFI when performed at one level, along with ABIs, can be billed with this code
93923	Noninvasive physiologic studies of upper or lower extremity arteries, multiple levels or with provocative maneuvers, <u>complete bilateral study</u> (segmental pressure, segmental Doppler, segmental PVR, segmental $TcPO_2$, with postural provocative maneuvers, with reactive hyperemia)	This code does not mean that all of the components need to be performed, but at least one of these tests at several levels on both limbs; it is important to note that if $TcPO_2$ is added to the normal protocol, it cannot be billed separately and in addition because it is considered part of the tests one can use!
93924	Noninvasive physiologic studies of lower extremity arteries, at rest and following treadmill stress testing, <u>complete bilateral study</u>	Here again the code includes a full test at rest (whatever your protocol may be) *and* retest after exercise; therefore, 93923 cannot be billed with this code
93925	Duplex scan of lower extremity arteries or arterial bypass grafts, <u>complete bilateral study</u>	This code is rather straightforward and involves duplex scan without any physiologic testing; therefore, if your protocol includes ABI with graft surveillance, you would be able to add 93922 to this code for billing (as specified above)

CPT Codes	Official Description	Appropriate Use and Restrictions
93926	Duplex scan of lower extremity arteries or arterial bypass grafts, <u>limited or unilateral study</u>	If the patient has grafts in both legs, never bill two of these; instead, use 93925; if the patient has several grafts in the same extremity, then unfortunately you still have to use this code (93926)
93930	Duplex scan of upper extremity arteries or arterial bypass grafts, <u>complete bilateral study</u>	Same as for 93925
93931	Duplex scan of upper extremity arteries or arterial bypass grafts, <u>limited or unilateral study</u>	Same as for 93926

Extremities Venous

CPT Codes	Official Description	Appropriate Use and Restrictions
93965	Noninvasive physiologic studies of extremity veins, <u>complete bilateral study</u> (e.g., Doppler waveform analysis with responses to compression and other maneuvers, phleborheography, plethysmography)	Here the trick is not to read too much into the code; although we do perform maneuvers with duplex and use PWD, because the primary testing is imaging, the code 93965 *cannot* be used in conjunction with it; the code can *only* be used if you perform an isolated physiologic test as defined
93970	Duplex scan of extremity veins including responses to compression and other maneuvers, <u>complete bilateral study</u>	This is the code we use most often; however, be aware that it is the same code whether you are looking for DVT, superficial or deep valvular incompetence, or mapping for CABG or bypass. In addition, if you are looking for DVT and need to also map the GSV, you cannot bill this code twice in the same day on the same leg!
93971	Duplex scan of extremity veins including responses to compression and other maneuvers, <u>unilateral or limited</u>	The trick here is that ICAVL requires at least a PW Doppler waveform of the contralateral CFV when examining one leg for DVT, but it still counts only as a unilateral scan

Visceral

CPT Codes	Official Description	Appropriate Use and Restrictions
93975	Duplex scan of arterial inflow and venous outflow of abdominal, pelvic, or scrotal contents and/or retroperitoneal organs, <u>complete study</u>	This is the code you would use for a bilateral study of the flow (arterial and venous) of both kidneys (if the patient has only one kidney, then use the limited study code), if evaluating for mesenteric ischemia (which should include celiac, SMA, and IMA), or if looking at liver vasculature (portal, hepatic), testicular torsion, varicocele, etc.
93976	Same as above, <u>limited study</u>	If looking at a kidney transplant or liver transplant or evaluating just one kidney
93978	Duplex scan of the aorta, inferior vena cava, iliac vasculature, or bypass grafts, <u>complete study</u>	By experience, this code should be rarely used, even when looking for aortic aneurysm; the exam rarely allows for easy scan of all vessels and even less of the IVC but would be used for postendograft evaluation
93979	Same as above, <u>limited study</u>	Mostly used for detection of aortic aneurysm

(Continued)

CPT Codes	Official Description	Appropriate Use and Restrictions
Penile		
93980	Duplex scan of arterial inflow and venous outflow of penile vessels, <u>complete study</u>	Rather straight forward code, except if you are also looking at scrotum for testicular torsion
93981	Same as above, <u>limited study</u>	
Dialysis		
93990	Duplex scan of hemodialysis access (including arterial inflow, body of access, and venous outflow)	This code cannot be used for routine exam, except at 6 months after the procedure to evaluate the maturation of the graft; however, it can be used for follow-up with specific clinical indicator or ICD-9 codes, such as difficult cannulation, thrombus aspiration, prolonged bleeding, pain at site, persistent swelling, and suspected low flow. It also cannot be used with any of the other codes for extremities unless these are billed for totally different reasons than the evaluation of predialysis access.
G0365	Vessel mapping prior to placement or creation of an autogenous hemodialysis conduit; includes arterial inflow and venous outflow	This code cannot be used on the same day 93971 is used (unless used for another reason than mapping), with another imaging technique, or on a limb that already has a dialysis access; it can only be used twice a year. Tip: Use G0365 in any limb that has not received any surgery and is being evaluated prior to placement of hemodialysis; otherwise, use 93971/93970.
Other		
76936	Ultrasound-guided compression repair of an arterial pseudoaneurysm or an arteriovenous fistula; this code includes the ultrasound evaluation by duplex, the ultrasound-guided compression, and the postcompression imaging by ultrasound; it is an example of a bundle code	Requires *direct* physician supervision (meaning physician must be present in the room)
76937	Ultrasound guidance for vascular access requiring evaluation of potential access site, documentation of selected vessel patency, concurrent real-time visualization of needle entry, with permanent recording and reporting	This code would be used, for example, if the access to the femoral artery was difficult before a cardiac catheterization or if the cannulation of the internal jugular vein was difficult; this seems to be the best code to use also for thrombin injection for pseudoaneurysm (the injection itself is billed under 36002)
76942	Ultrasonic guidance for needle placement (e.g., biopsy, aspiration, injection, localization device), imaging supervision, and interpretation	This code seems to fit also for the first portion of the previously described code, if placement of the needle is the only process required, meaning that time is not really spent looking at the patency of the vessel per se!

CPT Codes	Official Description	Appropriate Use and Restrictions
36475	Endovenous ablation therapy of incompetent vein, extremity, inclusive of all imaging guidance and monitoring, percutaneous, radiofrequency; first vein treated	
36476	Same as above, plus second and subsequent veins treated in a single extremity, each through separate access sites	Use 36475 and 36476 together only if testing and treating multiple veins
36478	Same as 36475 except that technique is laser (i.e., first vein treated)	
36479	Same as 36476 except that technique is laser (i.e., second and other veins treated using separate access sites)	Use 36478 and 36479 together only if testing and treating multiple veins
G0389	Ultrasound B-scan and/or real-time visualization with image documentation for abdominal aortic aneurysm screening	The patient needs to meet Medicare requirements according to SAAAVE Bill (male over 65 years old with history of smoking, or anyone, females included, with family history); this is a one-time exam as part of the "Welcome to Medicare" physical exam

PART II: Test Validation/Correlation Analysis

Measurement	Definition	Meaning
Sensitivity TP/TP + FN	Measures the ability of a test to detect disease when a disease is present. It is measured against a gold standard for the condition. It is calculated by dividing the number of true positive tests by all positive tests by gold standard.	Measures the validity of the test (that is a way to ensure the test actually measures what it is intended to measure). It is the probability of testing positive if the disease is truly present. As it increases, the number of people "missed" by the test will decrease.
Specificity TN/FP + TN	Measures the ability of a test, against a gold standard, to identify normal results and exclude disease. It is calculated by dividing the number of true negative tests by all negative tests by gold standard.	Measures the validity of the test. It is the probability of testing negative when the disease is truly absent. As it increases, the number of people "misdiagnosed" as having the disease or condition will decrease.
Accuracy TP + TN/TP + FP + FN + TN	Expresses the percentage of all exams (true positive and true negative) correctly identified by the test. It is calculated by dividing the number of true negative tests + true positive tests by the total number of exams evaluated.	This number always falls between the sensitivity and specificity, as well as between the PPV and NPV.
Positive Predictive Value (PPV) TP/TP + FP	Expresses the percentage of abnormal tests also abnormal by gold standard. It is calculated by dividing the number of true positive tests by the number of all positive tests.	Measures the probability that a person actually has the disease or condition given that he/she had a positive test. The more specific the test, the less likely that a person with a positive test will be free of disease and, therefore, the greater the PPV.
Negative Predictive Value (NPV) TN/FN + TN	Expresses the percentage of normal tests that are also normal by gold standard. It is calculated by dividing the number of true negative tests by the number of all negative tests.	Measures the probability that a person is truly disease or condition free given that the test is negative. The more sensitive the test, the less likely the person with a negative test will have the disease and, therefore, the greater the NPV.

Abbreviations: FN, false negative; FP, false positive; TN, true negative; TP, true positive.

The PPV can only be increased by increasing the specificity or by increasing the prevalence of the condition in the population under investigation. With rare diseases, the PPV will be low despite a high sensitivity and specificity.

	Number of Positive Tests by Gold Standard	Number of Negative Tests by Gold Standard
Number of Positive Tests by Methods Investigated (that would be your test)	True positive (TP)	False positive (FP)
Number of Negative Tests by Methods Investigated	False negative (FN)	True negative (TN)

Correlation analysis for the purpose of quality assurance allows you to test "your test." This means that you want to ensure your test leads to a similar conclusion for the same patient if/when applying another technique defined as a "gold standard." A "gold standard" is assumed to give a 100% (or close to) reliability to detect disease or its absence. However a "gold standard" is not always available.

Following is a table summarizing what test you can use for correlation and how to use the test for correlation in order to develop a quality assurance program for tests performed in vascular laboratories.

Noninvasive Tests	Test to Use for Correlation	How to Use Test for Correlation
Duplex Veins		
	Venogram	Build a correlation matrix (see below)
	Other noninvasive test such as APG	Build a correlation matrix
	Rescan option	Have another technologist repeat the study you just performed and compare results (can be done on one patient per week for example)
	Reinterpretation option	Select several studies and have them reinterpreted by another physician and then compare results
	Outcome study	Select positive and some negative studies and track results of follow-up scans; correlate with patient treatment, resolution of symptoms, other ancillary tests such as VQ scan, etc.
Physiologic Test for Veins		
	All above options are applicable here too, but using Duplex for rescan would be the easiest option	Build a correlation matrix
Physiologic Test for Peripheral Arteries		
	Angiogram	Build a correlation matrix for severity and location of disease
	MRA/CTA	Same as above
	Duplex	Same as above
	Angiogram	Build a correlation matrix for location of disease
	MRA/CTA	Same as above

(Continued)

Noninvasive Tests	Test to Use for Correlation	How to Use Test for Correlation
Duplex Abdominal or Cerebral Vasculature		
	Angiogram	Build a correlation matrix
	MRI or MRA	Same as above
	CT or CTA	For aneurysmal disease, CT is the best test for correlation; correlate for size and anatomic location

Example Correlation Matrix for Carotid Duplex Versus Angiogram

Duplex/Angiogram	Normal	0–15%	16–49%	50–79%	80–99%	Occluded
Normal	3					
0–15%	1	5				
16–49%		2	10	1		
50–79%				15		
80–99%				1	7	1
Occluded					1	3

Total exams: 50
Agreement for all categories: 43
Accuracy: 43/50 = 86%

	Positive by Gold Standard	Negative by Gold Standard
Positive by Duplex	40 (TP)	5 (FP)
Negative by Duplex	2 (FN)	3 (TN)

Sensitivity = 40/40 + 2 = 95%
Specificity = 3/3 + 5 = 37%
PPV = 40/40 + 5 = 89%
NPV = 3/3 + 2 = 60%

PART III: Comfort and Safety

In this section, my goal is to present what I would call "the ideal medicine cabinet" for the vascular lab. In this cabinet, I include items that, during the many years I spent in clinical settings, I learned can have a great impact on the serenity and efficiency of your daily work, although they may not have anything to do with the type of tests you need to perform and may thus not be available as standard (such as disposable gloves or sanitizing lotion).

I will not, however, engage in discussing the rules and regulations dictated by Occupational Safety and Health Administration (OSHA), Health Insurance Portability and Accountability Act (HIPAA), and so on, because these are or should be covered during orientation sessions for employment or presented in classes for students.

TABLE 1: **Patient's Comfort and Safety**

Items	Rationale
Cleaning supplies (soap, washcloths, and towels)	Accidents do happen! You may not always have the luxury of a fast-responding cleaning crew to help you wash a patient under some circumstances. It has happened to some of my patients in hospital or private office settings, and although the experience was not necessarily pleasant, it was important for the dignity of the patient.
Change of clothing	Keeping scrub suits of different sizes is a very important adjunct to the items described above. After cleaning a patient, he/she needs to be able to return home or on the hospital floor with dignity (which usually means with clothes on!).
Bag of adult diapers	Again, a great adjunct to the items described previously. Incontinence and advanced age are unfortunately not uncommon. After cleaning a patient and before redressing him/her, why not also prevent further accidents!
Source a fresh, drinkable water	Whether you live in a cold or warm climate, having a patient with a dry throat and trying to perform a carotid study, for example, can add to the challenge of an exam. Stop, offer a glass of water (if not contraindicated for inpatients particularly), and resume your test, which may become much easier!
Juices or candies	Patients suffering from diabetes mellitus are unfortunately a large portion of the population referred to vascular laboratories. Although most diabetics will be prepared and have the supplies they need to control or offset adverse events, a day in the doctor's office or a testing facility may be longer than anticipated. A glass of juice or a candy may make help offset hypoglycemia. This is only recommended for outpatient labs. For inpatients, a consultation with the nurse should precede any interventions.
Blanket and/or "booty" socks	These items have helped me tremendously in making any physiologic study easier. There is nothing more frustrating than trying to perform a physiologic test when the patient is cold and has constricted digital arteries. Aside from that, we should also remember that even if the temperature of a room is controlled for comfortable working conditions, a patient will be partially undressed and immobile for a test and therefore more susceptible to feel cold.

TABLE 2: **Your Comfort and Safety**

Items	Rationale
Change of clothing	For the accidents that do happen (as mentioned earlier) and because they may partially or completely "spill over" onto you.
Comfortable shoes	This is particularly important for those working in cold climate! I lived for 20 + years in Boston, and although wearing snow boots outside is a must in the winter, wearing snow boots all day while working in an overheated lab is very uncomfortable. I quickly learned to keep a pair of sneakers or clogs at work!
Altoid or mint tablet	This item was recommended by one of my students whose previous career was in a forensic pathology lab! Her advice to be able to handle any unwelcome (yet often uncontrollable) unpleasant odors is to place a mint tablet on your tongue and let it dissolve slowly throughout the exam to let your olfactory receptors time to get used to the ambient smells.
Items	Rationale
Disposable masks	These are recommended as much for your safety as for the safety of your patient. Our patients suffer from colds and so do we. Sometimes taking a day off is not possible, and some of our patients will have a depressed immune system. Why expose ourselves or others to a cold? Wear a mask or offer one to your patient.
Hand lotion	Standard precautions call for frequent hand washing and wearing disposable gloves, and both can induce and/or worsen dry skin. A bottle of hand lotion on the sink will help keep your skin healthy and prevent cracks (which can become a route of entry for pathogens).

TABLE 3: **Technical Help**

Items	Rationale

Bandage scissors

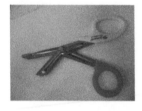

Some of our patients will present with bandages "inconveniently" located where we need to place a transducer to scan the appropriate vessel. Removing some bandages, particularly those used for venous ulcers, can be difficult. Bandage scissors are specifically designed to fit between the skin and the bandage without risks to the patient. Caution: Before removing any bandage, consult with the treating physician and/or nurse for the removal and appropriate care after removal. When working in a private office, we always had replacements for all types of wound dressings, so that when removal was warranted for the exam, I or the medical assistant could replace the dressing.

Sterile scanning pads

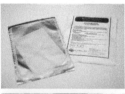

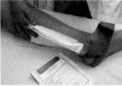

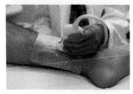

These are thin layers of congealed gel material presented in sterile packaging. If it is necessary to remove a wound dressing for scanning purposes, these are a must. The package needs to be opened using sterile technique, and the sterile part is placed over the entire wound before scanning. These pads prevent contamination of open wounds.

Plastic wrap

Refers to the rolls sold in supermarket for wrapping food or other items. This is a very useful item in any lab. I have used this on patients with cellulitis or other skin infections before placing blood pressure cuffs. Although I do disinfect cuffs regularly, and particularly after doing a test on patients with the ailments described previously, wrapping the limb with plastic offers an additional layer of protection for the patient and the cuff and did not deter from or affect the results of the test.

Gauze

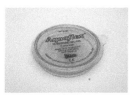

I sometimes use a thin layer of gauze for extra padding and comfort before placing the plastic wrap as explained above.

Stand-off pads

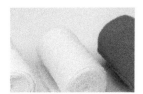

These are usually about ½ inch thick congealed gel pads and are very useful for scanning the anastomosis (at the wrist) of a Brescia-Cimino dialysis access or any other very superficial structures, such as the distal anastomosis of a lower extremity arterial bypass graft when placed at the dorsalis pedis artery.

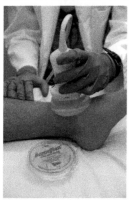

Double-sided tape

This item is useful to keep photoplethysmography (PPG) leads in place on the digits, particularly when used for monitoring flow with thoracic outlet syndrome maneuvers or Allen's test.

Surgical tape (hypoallergenic)

This item is very versatile and easily found in a hospital or outpatient setting and can be used to secure PPG leads or gauze, among many other uses.

Measuring tape

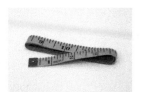

This item is often underrepresented in labs but very useful in many circumstances. I have used it to estimate the length of a superficial vein to be used for bypass graft, to measure the distance from a specific landmark (usually the knee or inguinal area) to an area of stenosis, and to measure the size of a limb, among many other uses.

Extra pillow

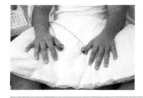

As demonstrated in the photo, a pillow can have many uses (if you do not have the latest, most ergonomic examination table!). It is particularly good for stabilizing the hands when PPGs are applied to the digits (we all know that PPGs are very sensitive sensors and any movement, even subtle, can induce "unreadable" waveforms).

Items	Rationale

Bucket

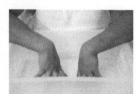

Although labs have sinks, I found that using a bucket filled with cold water for cold immersion studies is better for the patient's comfort.

Hand-held Doppler

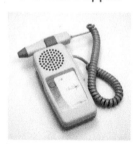

This item and the following one (sphygmomanometer) are useful when technical problems arise and the day needs to continue (it allows you to at least get data to calculate ABI); these are also useful in the inpatient setting because they are portable.

Sphygmomanometer

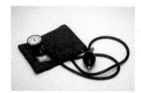

Same as above

Velcro

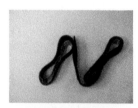

Velcro is a very versatile product. It can be used to hold a PPG lead in place. I have also used it to keep all my pressure cuffs easily accessible for a test and for cleaning (by placing the Velcro on the wall or a mounting board).

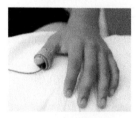

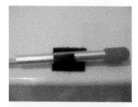

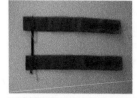

Transducer cleaner and disinfectant

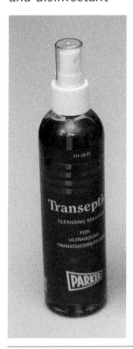

These products come in sprays and wipes. Before purchasing any particular brand, follow the guidelines for the equipment you have in the lab. These guidelines are usually in the user/technical manual.

Tourniquet

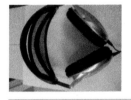

Although it is just a long and wide rubber band, a tourniquet can be used in the vascular lab with a slightly looser application than for phlebotomy, as an aid during measurement of superficial veins before harvest for graft conduit and to show measurement under maximum dilatation. Not a must but a nice adjunct.

Headphones

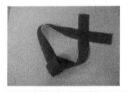

Every physiologic testing equipment and hand-held Doppler device has an adapter for headphones. This will serve two main purposes. For you, it will isolate you from background noise and let you concentrate on the Doppler signals. For the patient, it will make the test more peaceful because he/she will not have to listen to the Doppler or static (which can be very loud and disturbing to untrained ears).

Protection pads for bedding

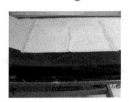

A handy and versatile adjunct to the "medicine cabinet"

Step stool

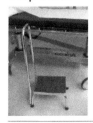

Models with a handlebar can serve several purposes. The primary purpose is to assist patients to move onto the examination table, the second is to be a resting step for the leg during an examination of the superficial veins for valve incompetence, and the third is to help a patient keep his/her balance when doing toe raises for lower extremity exercise.

Index